Advance Praise

"This important book is based on Dr. Devaki Lindsey Berkson's in-depth study of the science behind sexuality, gender expression, and brain power. It's an engaging read and is sure to be controversial."

—Patricia Johnson & Mark Michaels, Co-authors: *Partners in Passion, Great Sex Made Simple: Tantric Tips to Deepen Intimacy & Heighten Pleasure*, and *The Essence of Tantric Sexuality*

"Dr. Berkson and I have been life long friends. I know she translates excellent science into excellent advice and now she does it surrounding intimacy. A great read.

—Alan R. Gaby, M.D., Author of *Nutritional Medicine*

"I couldn't put this book down. *SEXY BRAIN* is a must read for anyone searching for a healthier lifestyle. Dr. Berkson writes in a simple yet elegant style. It is impossible for anyone to reach their optimal health or achieve rewarding sex without hormonal balance. Dr. Berkson's book provides all the information needed to understand why hormonal balancing and an active sex life are so important."

—David Brownstein, M.D., Author of 12 books, including *The Miracle of Natural Hormones* and *Dr. Brownstein's Natural Way to Health* Newsletter

"Dr. Berkson's latest book *SEXY BRAIN* is her newest masterpiece to add to her impressive list of books. As always, Dr. Berkson picks a topic of current interest, researches it to the finest detail and then compiles her findings in a logical, scientific, poetic, and easy-to-read format. Compared to other books on the topic, which seem to be little more than R-rated fiction, *SEXY BRAIN* takes the reader through a scientifically-backed journey into the human brain's role in physical attraction, emotional involvement, and the pleasures of intimacy. And the benefits. Even as a gynecologist, I had no idea that intimacy and lovemaking were so brain protective! This is a must read for any professional who counsels patients or anyone who simply wants to get more out of intimacy and the physical pleasures that life has to offer."

—Jack Monaco, M.D., Nashville, TN, Gynecologist and Professor of Functional Medicine

"In the first six pages I was already blown away! People are going to love this! What I also appreciate is that this is such a well-written book that parents, with complete peace of mind, can gift it to their young adult kids to learn all the in's and out's of intimacy and how to make marriages last."

—Carol L. Roberts, M.D., author, *Good Medicine: A Return to Common Sense*, Naples, Florida

"My sex life with my husband was already great, but after reading Dr. Berkson's book, *SEXY BRAIN,* our sex life has now climbed to a higher, better level. After doing the exercises in the book, we unleashed the frequency of my orgasms one after the other. Dr. Lindsey's book will not only revolutionize your sex life but it also will change the way you view orgasms as they relate to your health. Her incredible way of incorporating the medical info with the pleasurable side of intimacy provides a provocative read. I would feel good about giving my son this book when he gets engaged."

—Tanjie Brewer, CEO of the COVE [Community for Women to Achieve Vitality, Health and Style], Chicago, IL

"I could not put it down. I am very, very impressed by how well Berkson writes. Her degree of research and her extraordinary writing style are impressive. This is wonderful work and I regard Berkson as having proven herself to be an authority on this important topic."

—Bob Steinberg, CEO, Sage Manufacturing, Carmel Valley, CA

"I have read all of Berkson's books, and that's a lot, and I keep them on my shelf as references for female health and nutrition. Berkson's new book combines scholarly facts with humor and insight. Rather than sit on a shelf, it's my new bedside companion!"

—Bee Zollo, Hospice RN, Santa Fe, NM

"This work is BRILLIANT. Berkson talking about the gut as it relates to love and sex is really something! I did not know about the connection between testosterone and lungs. You make leaps and jumps that are really fresh, new, and exciting. It is all done with a lot of love—and to help people love each other. Your work is really inspired. I don't want to take hormone replacement myself, but it doesn't matter. There is so much else to grab onto."

—Judith Fein, author of *Life is a Trip*, *The Spoon from Minkowitz*, *Huffington Post* and *Psychology Today* Blogger, & Ted Talk presenter

"Dr. Berkson, thank you for writing such a fascinating, informative, and easy to understand book. I learned more from your book on how hormones run my life and bedroom than from years of visits to many doctors' offices from Oklahoma to California. All men and women wanting successful relationships and vibrant brain health should read this book."

—Brenda Johnson, Grateful Homemaker, Tulsa, OK

"The topic of safe hormones and intimacy is so crucial to overall health, this book deserves to be read by everyone who is concerned about their brain, sex life, and the future health of her children. Dr. Berkson is a nutritional and hormonal visionary who blends science with substance. Now she artfully adds "sex" to that mix."

—Ann Louise Gittleman, PhD, CNS, Award Winning New York Times bestselling author of *The New Fat Flush Plan*

Also By D. Lindsey Berkson

Books on Hormones, Health, and Digestion

The Foot Book
Hormone Deception
Healthy Digestion The Natural Way
Hormones Made Easy
Hormones Aren't Gorillas
Natural Answers for Women's Health Questions
Safe Hormones, Smart Women
Nutritional Gastroenterology
Body, Mind, Hormones Mission eBook
Retraining Your Tongue
My Mother Who Wore Her Purse As a Shoe
Herman The Vegetarian Cat (a coloring book)

As Contributing Author
Body, Mind & Spirit
Alternative Medicine: The Definitive Guide
Reviving Mr. Happy

Other Books

Juicy Souls
Why It's So Hard To Keep All Our Ducks in a Row
Why Is Love So Hard
Crossing The Bridge
HeartSpeak
What The Universe Wants From Us Is Absolutely Nothing

SEXY BRAIN

Sizzling Intimacy & Balanced Hormones Prevent
Alzheimer's, Cancer, Depression & Divorce

Dr. Devaki Lindsey Berkson

Our Intimacy And Cognition Are Under Attack
Learn How Sex Can Save Them

Awakened Medicine Press
Austin, TX

Sexy Brain
Sizzling Intimacy & Balanced Hormones Prevent Alzheimer's, Cancer, Depression & Divorce
By Dr. Devaki Lindsey Berkson

Published by Awakened Medicine Press, Austin, Texas

Paperback: ISBN 13: 978-0-9973661-0-5

Cover Design/Graphics: Rosita Alvarez www.RositaAlvarez.com
Interior Design: Karrie Ross www.karrieross.com
Editor: Barbara Markus
Cover Photo: Elaine McDaniel

Publisher's Cataloging-In-Publication Data
(Prepared by The Donohue Group, Inc.)

Names: Berkson, Lindsey.
Title: Sexy brain : sizzling intimacy & balanced hormones prevent Alzheimer's,
    cancer, depression & divorce / Dr. Devaki Lindsey Berkson.
Description: Austin, Texas : Awakened Medicine Press, [2017] | Includes bibliographi-
    cal references and index.
Identifiers: LCCN 2017930434 | ISBN 978-0-9973661-0-5 (paperback) | ISBN 978-
    0-9973661-1-2 (mobi) | ISBN 978-0-9973661-2-9 (ePub)
Subjects: LCSH: Sexual health. | Sex—Health aspects. | Libido—Health aspects. |
    Hormones, Sex. | Detoxification (Health) | Gastrointestinal system.
Classification: LCC RA788 .B47 2017 (print) | LCC RA788 (ebook) | DDC 613.9—
    dc23

Dedication

To all those who have not yet experienced "awakened intimacy" or mind-protective sex and doubt they even exist, when actually it's nature's strategy to keep us healthy, happy, and cognitively fit.

Table Of Contents

Part 1
You are Designed To Have Frequent and Fabulous Sex

Part 2
How To Do It So Your Brain And Partner Love It

Foreword By Pamela W. Smith, MD

Dr. Devaki Lindsey Berkson is a gem! We officially met on a phone call about five years ago while I was doing research for a seminar where I teach other healthcare providers the nuances of functional and metabolic medicine. One of my presentations was supported by some of the outstanding research that Devaki has made her "modus operandi." Her work is stellar as anyone fortunate enough to call her a colleague will attest to. I am enriched and truly blessed that Lindsey's path has intersected mine.

Her previous books have "connected the dots" and have shown us the incredible importance that the nexus of hormone health, gut health, and environmental toxins plays in our lives every day. She has done this with clarity, without confusing "science-speak", making her work logical, entertaining, and accessible to everyone. It is clear that her primary focus is healthy patients.

In her latest book, Dr. Berkson has done it again. Her words flow effortlessly as she "connects the dots" in a way only she can. She clearly demonstrates that the great communication that can lead to a great sex life, indeed, actually begins at the atomic level! Devaki demonstrates that this communication is truly a two way street: healthy and balanced hormone levels lead to sex, which, in turn, leads to healthy hormone levels! We also learn that men and women, even though they share the same hormones (just in differing amounts) are truly wired in amazingly different and complimentary ways due to our basic chemistry. Our "give and take" relationships are molecular in origin and essential to our mental, physical, and spiritual well-being.

But all of this fascinating information so well laid out by Dr. Berkson would be academic if not for her insightful and practical suggestions on how to initiate these connections that benefit our sexiest organ, the brain. Sprinkled throughout the book, Berkson offers nuggets of wisdom keeping us riveted and eagerly turning the pages.

This latest book of hers should not be considered just another "brick in the wall" of what we call a healthy lifestyle, but rather, an important cornerstone to a life well lived. Read on, learn things, and be amazed.

—Pamela W. Smith, M.D., MPH, MS

Dr. Pamela W. Smith is the author of eight best-selling books, including her latest: *What You Must Know About Thyroid Disorders*.

Foreword By Jonathan V. Wright, MD

Our ancestors knew that sex at all ages is good for us in many ways. But in our "scientific age," many physicians, professors, researchers, and others refuse to believe something unless it can be "proven" scientifically. Fortunately, science has now caught up and proven this concept with hundreds of research studies. We're fortunate that Dr. Berkson has taken the time to gather and read that science and explain it so understandably well in this book.

In SEXY BRAIN, Dr. Berkson uses her deep understanding of how sex relates to published brain and body science, telling us in understandable language how to improve our sex lives, and actually protecting and improving our health—especially brain health—by doing so. An excellent book with excellent information for our health and longevity, as well as happiness—if we act on the information it contains.

Hormone health is the foundation of great sex, intimacy, relationships, and families, but it often requires hormone replacement. If you read Dr. Berkson's last book, *Safe Hormones, Smart Women* (2010) and/or *Stay Young & Sexy with Bio-identical Hormone Replacement: The Science Explained* (2009), a book written by Lane Lenard Ph.D. and me, you'll find many more details about bioidentical hormone replacement and its role in intimacy and health.

Dr. Berkson shares with me a history and profound interest in hormones. She did her first rotation in integrative medicine with me (and with Dr. Alan Gaby, who was a student then, too). She appears to have "caught" the bioidentical hormone "bug" then.

In 1982, with the help of pharmacist Ed Thorpe, I was able to write the very first comprehensive bioidentical hormone prescriptions in these United States for a symptomatic menopausal woman. (Some say that makes me "the father of bioidentical hormone replacement," but bio-identical hormone replacement actually originated in China nearly a thousand years ago!)

The results were so good for her, and later for her friends—better memory and brain function, better libido and sex lives, as well as relief from menopausal symptoms—that some of these women urged their husbands to come in for their own hormone evaluations. Men being men, many of them focused first on their sex lives. I reminded them, as Dr. Berkson discusses in this book, that it was very likely that testosterone would significantly lower their risk of Alzheimer's disease or other cognitive decline, and that estrogen very likely would do the same for women. This was later proven to be a fact.

Why focus on preventing Alzheimer's disease and cognitive decline with bio-identical hormone replacement and not on sex life first? It's simple: For either a man or a woman, what does a sex life matter if we can't remember what we did and with whom? *Sexy Brain* is a great title: it says it all!

—Jonathan V. Wright MD

Tahoma Clinic
Tukwila, Washington
www.tahomaclinic.com

Foreword By Norman Shealy, MD PhD

SEXY BRAIN by Dr. Berkson provides terrific information for the most important life activity beyond having air, water, food, clothes and shelter! I am talking about intimacy.

Healthy people have healthy desire and abilities. Berkson shows in easy language the scientific basis for how the outer and inner environments are assaulting your most intimate desire and abilities. She then shows you what to do about it.

Two decades ago I did a study with four happily married couples. I measured blood levels of diverse hormones before and after sex. After three days of running the same tests, it was clear that intimacy boosts healthier hormone production.

Berkson shows how this hormone production boosts cognition. She shows that "awakened intimacy," as she calls it, from hugging to intercourse, is like getting a healthy jolt of hormone replacement for both men and women.

A huge percentage of people do not nurture their sexuality and their cognition is missing out.

I am a neurosurgeon, trained at Johns Hopkins. Years ago I became deeply aware of how energy, nutrition, and hormonal health are the authentic basis of getting well at the root level. I opened the only hospital wing in the U.S. based on nutrition and energy medicine that operated for 30 years.

I have a deep understanding that healthy intimacy, balanced hormones, and healthy nutrition contribute to great intimacy, healthier brains, and happier families.

SEXY BRAIN puts this all together in one book.

A great read that I highly recommend.

—C. Norman Shealy, M.D., Ph.D.

Founder and CEO, International Institute of Holistic
Medicine, Editor of Journal of Comprehensive Integrative
Medicine, Holos Energy Medicine Education Professor
Emeritus, Author of LIVING BLISS
 http://www.normshealy.com

Introduction

Sex is not frivolous. It's one of Mother Nature's designs to keep adults well, and to keep relationships and families stable. The idea that sex is as good for your health as it is for your pleasure is so new that few have the understanding or the exact tools to pull it off.

It turns out that satisfying, frequent sex, especially with someone you care for, respect, and with whom you have quality communication, is right up there with veggies and exercise, often giving better heart benefits than by consuming supposedly cardio-protective medications like statins. And gives better brain benefits than from doing crossword puzzles.

In fact, how the brain experiences intimacy is a very hot research topic now that we can look directly inside the brain with MRIs (magnetic resonance imaging) and see exactly what sex does to it. Brain imaging studies have looked inside male and female brains to see what is going on during sex with beloveds, with friends with benefits, or by oneself. It turns out that there are vastly diverse payoffs and big variations in how orgasms, the use of condoms, and relationship status turn on or off the brains of men versus women.

For years in the clinical trenches, I've seen that when sex lives are improved, *everything* gets better: physical health, emotional health, job performance, family and social dynamics. Even in 80- and 90-year-olds. But many of us have no clue what steps to take to achieve *awakened brain-gasms*—my terms for sex that boosts brains as well as systemic health. You will soon learn that the more often individuals make love, especially after 50 years of age, the better their cognition!

It is absolutely clear that we are meant to have incredible intimacy to maintain incredible health. Nature never does anything without a reason. Pleasure is meant to be part of our lives. This can mean touching and hugging, not necessarily intercourse, or it can be amazing sex steaming up the bedroom windows. The emphasis is on human *connection*. However, many patients admit in the privacy of my office that they merely tolerate sex for the sake of their mate. I hear this frequently, even from women and men in their 20s.

Just as science is proving the benefits of sex, there is a growing epidemic of diminished intimacy:

- The Public Health Agency of Sweden is studying the nation's bedroom habits because so many young Swedes are "doing it" less and enjoying it less.

- A massive UK survey revealed that young men and women, ages 16 to 21, had sexual dysfunctions similar to those mostly found in seniors.

- As the obesity epidemic grows, younger and mid-life males are becoming low in testosterone, fertility, and sex drive.

Our toxic world is attacking your hormones and happiness, even in young adults. Do you have any idea what to do about it?

Since I am a hormone scholar who has worked at an estrogen think tank associated with Tulane and its medical school; and since I have been working for over 40 years in the clinical and academic fields of how hormones run our bodies; and since I have self-healed the assaults from the deadliest hormonal medication my mother was given when pregnant with me and learned how to stop my tumor madness; and since I have designed the first science-based "receptor detox" to make hormones work no matter how toxic our environment has become...

I knew I had to write this book.

Great sex!

Everyone loves great sex (if they can achieve it). And science says that great sex loves us.

In 1981, I had the honor to practice functional medical/nutritional care in the very first integrative medical clinic in the U.S. in Palo Alto, California. The visionary cardiologist, Carl Ebnother MD, headed it. Dr. Ebnother was one of the first to add sex to the picture. On his prescription pads, Dr. E might write, "Have enjoyable sex three times a week," right next to a script for lowering blood pressure.

Dr. E taught me something I never forgot. He said, "The very first thing I try to figure out with each patient is their *will to live* versus their *will to die.* All the meds or nutrients in the world won't help anyone, especially their heart, if they don't have a greater will to live. Great sex makes that happen for many."

Most people these days think that when they fall in love with the "right" person, great sex will automatically follow. It's as if sitting in front of a grand piano could automatically morph you into an accomplished pianist. Great sex, like everything else, has to be learned. There should be no guilt in understanding that we need to have guidelines to achieve great sex and how to make it work for us in the most pleasurable, natural, and health-promoting ways. Great sex requires effective knowledge.

This book provides a complete, science-based, intimacy skill set.

You will learn that great sex leans on healthy hormones, which depend on nutrients and digestive health. The more our hormones, gut and nutrition are in sync, so is our sex life. Bet you didn't realize your gut was linked to your genitals.

You may long for romantic love and a dazzling mate, but have never been taught how to be a great lover. You may not have had the science explained to you as to why you should even aspire to be a great lover.

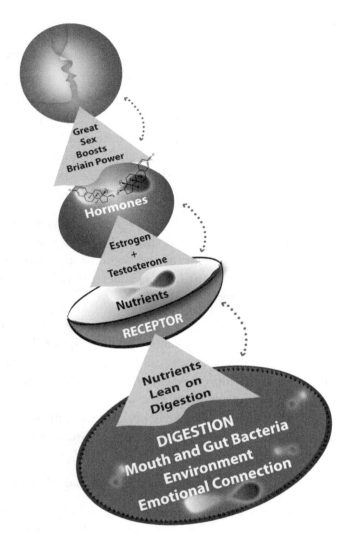

Up until now, scientists, doctors, and lay people have not known about the diverse benefits of sex, especially for our brain. And we have not understood that many of us don't achieve these benefits because we don't understand our differences and how to be with each other. Male and female perceptions, behaviors and expectations are hard-wired to be amazingly different, often creating huge obstacles to achieving great sex and all its gains. Grasping how very varied each other's atoms and molecules rule our attempts to make love and make love stay, guarantees being better lovers. I introduce this new *Hormone Language of Love*.

Welcome to the new world of the neurobiology of intimacy!

About this book

This book was officially birthed when I was asked to collaborate with a team of medical hormone specialists, along with Dr. Robert Ersek, a renowned surgeon, on a book about erectile dysfunction to be used in their new erectile dysfunction clinics.

While I was doing due diligence for this book, I came across a massive explosion of rigorous research on *sex science* that stunned me. I had already written over eight works on hormones, but I was frankly astonished at the number of elegant scientific trials demonstrating the benefits of healthy sex. Women having what they perceived to be *satisfying* sex used fewer antidepressants, made fewer suicide attempts, had a higher quality of life, and less plaque in their arteries; men had less cancer, heart disease, brain fog, and even better immune systems and gut health, which we now know is the mother of all health.

This book, written for both men and women, is based on 40 years of my clinical experience with thousands of patients and what they've told me about their sex lives, as well as the evidence-based scientific research.

You will be dumbfounded to learn that at the basic level of the atom, females are set up to *give* and males to *take*. In the language of orgasm neurology, female brains are set up to get more benefits by deeper sexual *satisfaction* while men get it from more *frequency*. This book gives you exact steps for dealing with these hard-wired differences.

And this book shows how sex serves:

Brain health. Sex boosts better cognition, cognitive reserve, and self-esteem. Not just by another notch-in-the-belt conquest kind of thing. It occurs through actual intimacy—hugging, touching, being present with each other, and intercourse—which then literally delivers optimizing signals to specific brain regions.

Relationship health. While writing this book, the Swedes came out with a groundbreaking study. It showed that daily sensuality and mutually satisfying sex keeps couples and families together. The government recommends that sex education should be part of premarital counseling.

Contemporary psychologists say people need three things to be happy: food, shelter, and intimacy. May this book give you and your mate responsible, health-promoting, brain-boosting, pleasure-filled intimacy, fostering truly happy relationships that are destined to succeed.

About the Author

Hormones—their science, clinical applications, and controversies—have been my life-long passion as well as my personal story. I lost a kidney, an adrenal gland, half my thyroid gland, 18 lymph nodes, and even more, in 15 major surgeries. But it was more than confusing as to why this was happening to me. From early on, I'd grown my own food and eaten a healthy plant-based diet. I was a robust athlete. I was doing everything right, but getting all the wrong outcomes. Why?

As I was writing *Hormone Deception* (McGraw-Hill 2000), one of the early breakthrough books on how everyday pollutants can mimic and damage our own hormones, I was shocked that many of the proven effects of endocrine disruptors had been happening to me. I immediately sent away for my mother's birth records and discovered, to my horror, that I was one of the very victims of the exact public health issue (endocrine disruption) that I was writing about.

My mother, like millions of other pregnant women for over 36 years, was given the most powerful synthetic estrogen ever invented (DES). It was prescribed like a prenatal vitamin! Now it's recognized as the most dangerous carcinogens ever invented. It was finally made illegal in 1971 (though it's still used in feedlots to fatten up cattle for lots of American burgers and steak).

I have endured the consequences of endocrine disruption—hormones gone bad—all my life. But I always say if you know what's wrong, you can fix it. By sleuthing through the research, I found that DES caused tumors by damaging protective tumor suppressor genes. When a cancer cell started to grow, I couldn't stop it. So I looked for what could. I figured out that safe metabolites of estrogen and even some foods could reboot these genes. I had a compounding pharmacy make up the first individualized hormone formula for me and I finally got well.

That started me on my 15-year journey of strategic use of safe hormones to help others become healthier and sexier.

Based on my research for *Hormone Deception*, I was invited to join *The Center for Bioenvironmental Research* at Tulane and Xavier Universities as a distinguished hormone scholar, one of the greatest honors of my life. There I worked with the top scientific hormone gurus. I had already formulated the first nutraceutical sold in the U.S. for menopause. I went on to co-patent a safe hormone replacement therapy and a medication for dialysis and kidney patients. I co-published original dialysis research with The University of Texas Health Science Center at Houston. I now teach continuing medical education courses on strategic hormones and nutrition to pharmacists, MDs, and other health professionals.

I have degrees in psychoneurobiology, communications, functional medicine, and nutrition. I consult with patients and physicians worldwide on hormones, gut health, and intimacy. Past books include a work on female health and hormones (*Natural Answers for Women's Health Questions*, Simon & Schuster 2002), the mind-body-nutrition link (*Healthy Digestion the Natural Way*, Wiley, 1998), and the science behind natural hormone therapy and its link to nutrition (*Safe Hormones, Smart Women*, Awakened Medicine 2010).

I lived in a spiritual community with Swami Satchidananda where I was certified as a meditation and yoga teacher. I took up dancing and for decades twirled around the globe. Yoga and dance are all about *connection*. So is great sex.

All these facets of my life, plus the research and books, now converge in your bedroom!

Click here for FREE Food-gasm recipe booklet from Dr. Berkson's kitchen. http://drlindseyberkson.com/sexybrain/

Go to SexyBrainSystem.com for more information.

SEXY
BRAIN

Our Intimacy And Cognition Are Under Attack
Learn How Sex Can Save Them

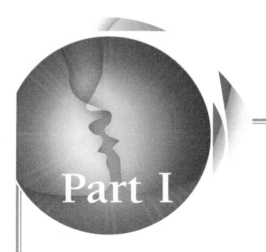

Part I

You Are
Designed
To Have
Frequent & Fabulous
Sex

CHAPTER 1

Hormone Love Language

*L*iz was a high-powered businesswoman, successful in every arena but the bedroom. Her husband, Sam, was her high school sweetheart. They'd been married for 25 years, but had fallen into the habit of leading separate lives and sleeping on separate sides of the bed.

Liz came in to see me because hot flashes were keeping her up at night and headaches were getting her down during the day. Many of her hormone levels tested low. A food evaluation exposed her to be a candy-a-holic. Sugar blocks hormone signals and her daily pain meds, NSAIDs, block them too.

Liz cleaned up her diet. She took specific nutrients and individualized hormone replacement. Within weeks she was sleeping like a rock, had tons more energy and no more headaches.

But what really blew her mind was how much her old sex drive woke up. She dragged Sam in. I explained how great sex supports cognition and vibrancy. Sam got motivated to eat better and get his hormones tested and treated. In a short time, Sam and Liz felt like they had when they first met. "Connection" came back. Their lives improved in body, mind and spirit. This is what healthy hormones can do for love.

Hormone Ergonomics

Hormones affect every area of your life. Not just sexy or reproductive issues, but every single part of you—your guts and brain as well as your libido.

To understand how hormones work, think of your body as having an internal Internet system. One cell tells another cell what to do. How? By email. What delivers most of this email? Hormones. Hormones send emails that tell cells all throughout your body (a wide swath of biological real estate, including the kidneys, heart, vocal chords, etc.) what to do to keep you alive and kicking.

But hormones also dictate *perception*. They have tremendous influence on how men and women see each other, and how they attempt to love and support each other. Or fail at it. Some men can stand in front of a gorgeous woman and feel nothing at all because their hormones aren't working right, and these days this is occurring in younger and younger men. And women.

Once you understand how profoundly hormones dictate your life, behavior, perceptions of reality, and even every aspect of wooing and sex, it will eliminate much of the frustration that often arises between men and women. Once you know how men and women are different at their biologic core, and how on every level the differences between estrogen and testosterone resonate into your neurology, psyche, bedroom, and therapist's office, you will *finally* have the tools you need to come together with your sexual partner in harmony and happiness rather than discord and disappointment.

Dr. Mary Carlson, an associate professor of neuroscience in psychiatry at Harvard Medical School, coined the term *liberation biology*. It refers to an "aha" moment when you figure out how something works inside your physical body, and this understanding leads to a larger understanding of the world around you.

Understanding something in your physiology and expanding that insight to larger themes in the rest of your life is an exciting concept.

I have found this to be the case with estrogen and testosterone, and their unique contribution to intimacy. So before diving headlong into the how-to's of sex, you have to have some understanding about hormones. (But if you just can't wait, turn to Chapters 12 and 13.)

. . .

You will see that estrogen is complex while testoterone is simpler.

. . .

You will see that estrogen is complex while testosterone is simpler. Therein lies the rub. You live these differences between estrogen and testosterone in your conversations and bedrooms. But if you really *get* them (the differences have to be embraced, not resisted), understand and digest them, you can learn to make the differences work *for* you in greater pleasure and mind-boosting sex.

Hormone ergonomics

You get frustrated. All you want is pleasure and love and instead you get harshness in your relationship, in the bedroom, and even in trying to hold a real conversation. Why? Hormonal "is-ness."

Men and women have the same hormones but in different ratios, and these hormones pull powerfully on our biology and mating practices. So to learn how they act differently is to become a wiser person and a much wiser lover.

Each hormone has a specific set of personality traits that come from how its atoms and molecules are shaped. Nature is a master shape-shifter, and shapes affect you in ancient and haunting ways. Plus, each hormone has its own physiologic set of interactions and rhythms. These hormonal personalities reverberate into the personalities of men and women and up into the bedroom.

What is a hormone?

Hormones are signaling or "speaking" molecules. The body functions through "physiological conversations." This means that the "words" are actually chemical signals that are delivered to cells, like an *internal* biological Internet system. In the same way that an email delivers information to you, hormones deliver "emails" or signals to cells telling them what to do.

The ultimate job of hormones is to get their email messages delivered to the genes that are deep inside cells. Genes contain all our genetic information, but to work they need to be turned "on" or "off." Hormonal signals direct genes to turn on or off, which tells the cells what to do, when to do it, and how long to do it for. And your life unfolds. And sex sizzles.

Hormone receptors

Hormones start their message delivery service by docking into hormone receptors. So hormones are a two-part system: first, a *hormone* and second, the *receptor* it delivers signals to. You gotta have both! Receptors are proteins shaped like satellite dishes, ready to receive hormonal input. Hormones dock inside the receptors. The shape of the individual hormone merges with the shape of the satellite receptor and they shape-shift, like two people hugging under a sheet rolling around making love. This movement is *molecular shimmying*. This is the hormone sending its signals to the genes.

Receptors receive a hormone signal. They translate that signal to the gene. This chatting results in hormone/receptor shimmering. In response, you have *libido, focus, motivation, and a zip in your step.* All these signals make you who you are, both in and out of the bedroom. And, as major signals of life are based on shapes and shape-shifting, this is why all of us are so deeply touched by "shape" itself—the shape of a mountain range on the horizon or the curve of your lover's lips and hips.

Receptors line cells, inside and out, and are uniquely designed to receive and translate emails that *any* hormone (estrogen, testosterone, adrenal hormones, thyroid hormones, insulin, and even vitamin D) intends to deliver. They shape-shift and signal. Both men and women have a total of 48 such receptors, some are still being discovered or are yet unknown.

Much of the time, each specific hormone delivers emails to its own exact receptors. For example, the female hormone *estrogen* delivers messages to specific *estrogen receptors*. The male hormone *testosterone* delivers messages to specific *testosterone receptors*. Thyroid hormone delivers messages to thyroid receptors, and so on.

However, good hormonal intentions can get thwarted. Emails can get hijacked. Some young men have low testosterone levels, and thus low libido and performance skills, because pollutants or stress are clogging and bogging down their receptors. Many women wear toxic cosmetics or eat too much sugar or drink too many alcoholic cocktails, which cause hormonal imbalances and a non-functioning Internet system. These days, you even can be in your twenties or thirties and suffer from hormonal imbalance that's sabotaging your sexual well-being.

Hormones are complex and there are many complexities possible in how, when, and where they deliver their emails. But for our purposes here, a basic understanding of the signaling process is all you need.

Simple testosterone

Even though it's known as the male hormone, both men and women have the hormone testosterone and testosterone receptors.

Testosterone is a molecule with very specific functions that we have come to think of as "manly." For example, testosterone delivers emails to the male prostate, penis, and sperm to make them function optimally. But testosterone also delivers emails to *any* and *all* cells that have testosterone receptors in both men and women.

Testosterone receptors line the scrotum in men and breast tissue in women. But cells not related to sexual or reproductive tissues, like the gut and the brain, also have testosterone receptors. There are testosterone receptors throughout the entire body, including the heart, bones, lungs, and skin. Signals to all these cells can affect energy, libido, motivation, and mood in both men and women. When you make love, even when you cuddle, testosterone signals can be sent to all these tissues. This is a good thing.

Researchers at Harvard have recently identified testosterone receptors in gut bacteria as well as along the digestive track. So testosterone, the male hormone in both men and women, and gut bacteria in both genders, help keep each other healthy and libido soaring.

Testosterone signaling protects a tiny set of cells in the brain that is our "physical soul"—the seat of our memories and the sense of who we are. It is called the *hippocampus*. You will learn that making love nudges your hippocampus and thinking abilities healthward!

.   .   .

Maleness "protects" femaleness.

.   .   .

Testosterone delivers emails to receptors in the heart that keep the basic heart cells (cardiomyocytes) living longer in both women and men.

Testosterone is broken down into smaller parts (metabolites) that protect breast cells in women from turning into breast cancer cells. In this way, *maleness* "protects" *femaleness* as nature intended.

Sex boosts testosterone

As you can see, both men and women thrive on appropriate levels of testosterone. Testosterone is so crucial to both men and women that nature has set it up so that *making love increases testosterone* levels in both men and women.

The Department of Psychology at Georgia State University tested this. They had four heterosexual couples make love over eleven nights.

Testosterone levels were measured before and after sex.

- Testosterone levels *increased* every night when there was intercourse,

- And *decreased* when there was none.

This pattern was *exactly the same* for males and females. The scientists concluded that sexual activity gently and healthfully promotes a boost in testosterone. This is good thing for Venus and Mars and their brains and self-esteem.

Nature's tactics. This part of sex is fundamental but has not been appreciated until now. Nature is waste not, want not. She does not do anything in the human body without deliberate reasons. Nature knows we will mate. She wants us to mate. And the intention is for the human brain to continue to have a good chance at being healthy gray matter for as long as it can. Sex, you see, is part of that plan.

Male hormones, called *androgens*, signal the *androgen receptor*. Besides testosterone, other male-acting hormones (DHEA, DHT, and others) come from the adrenal gland or are breakdown metabolites of testosterone itself. So the male hormone family has testosterone as the major go-to player, with four to five other male-acting molecular players.

And making love boosts these healthy male signals in *both* men and women.

Complex Estrogen

Estrogen, the main female hormone, is more complex than testosterone. Sir Henry Hallett Dale was a knight, scientist, physiologist, and physician who shared a Nobel Prize on nerve research. Dr. Dale was famous for his in-depth know-how surrounding all things estrogen. Sir Dr. Dale gave a famous talk at the Society for Endocrinology in the 1960s, only years before his death, on the extraordinary personality of estrogen. He said that if he were discussing the discovery of simpler hormones, like insulin or adrenaline, his story would be short. But, Sir Dale admitted with a sigh, "Everything surrounding estrogen is a whole tumultuous tangle of threads," illustrating that estrogen is the most complex hormone of all hormones.

Most doctors and even science books regard *estradiol* as the major estrogen, with only two other estrogen players—*estrone* and *estriol*. But biologically, estrogen is much more elaborate. The word *estrogen* is actually not just one hormone, but an umbrella term for up to *sixty* slightly different types of estrogenic molecules, meaning they all have some kind of estrogen-like action. They can all deliver estrogen signals, yet these signals can be extremely different from each other.

Estrogen signals have been around a long long time. She was the first sex hormone signal on earth. Estrogen has been sending signals in coral reefs and early organisms for over 400 million years. She's the oldest, strongest, loudest, and most complex hormone on the planet.

Neither sex would thrive for long if they didn't both have adequate blood levels of estrogen. Just as men and women both need testosterone, they both also need estrogen. Estrogen sends emails to cells to boost functioning of the heart, blood vessels, gut, bones, skin, lungs, sexual organs, kidneys, vocal chords, and, most of all, the brain.

Estrogen in the brain

Both estrogen and testosterone "feed" the human brain.

Estrogen sends signals to estrogen receptors in the brain, spinal chord, and in the gut and gut wall. Estrogen protects nerves and nerve-signaling molecules (called *neurotransmitters*) that help the brain in the head, as well as in the second "brain" in the gut, to function optimally.

In both genders, estrogen also helps keep the *hippocampus* healthy. The hippocampus is robustly lined with receptors for *both* estrogen and testosterone. Studies tracking hormone levels with cognition as we age are showing that hormones protect brain health across a life span. And the more we make love, especially pleasure-filled intimacy, even just the act of touching, holding, and cuddling (especially in women), the more exposure we get to these brain protective hormones.

Brain Shape

You are a product of the *shape* of your brain. The better the shape, the better the function. As you age, all of you shrinks. This is easy to see with your skin, but not with your brain. But after the age of 25, your brain very slowly starts to shrink as your hormones start to decline. Your brain shape alters and brain function sputters. This brain aging picks up speed in your forties and onward. There are protective actions you can take. A healthy lifestyle, exercise, and eating several fish meals a week all help to keep your brain in better shape. But the best brain shaper protectors of all are keeping your *hormones balanced* and your sex life *regular* and *satisfying*!

With magnetic resonance imaging (MRI) we can look right into the brain and identify the size of the hippocampus. The psychiatric department at McGill University did just this. They measured "shrunken" hippocampi in aging men and women and then gave their brain cells "food" in the form of hormone replacement. Follow-up imaging showed that these precious cells re-volumized back to a more youthful shape. This effect was accomplished rapidly, within four to five weeks. Most importantly, at the same time, these elders got back their memory, focus, confidence, and mojo.

This research was so elegant it won the coveted Kurt Richer Award of 2008 and the McGill laboratory was awarded $100,000. This revolutionary brain imaging study clearly demonstrated that hormones, which the body naturally makes, when given as replacement, keep the brain young. Hormones can "anti-age" the brain.

.   .   .

So the big "O" is actually Mother Nature's way to boost these hormones in both men and women.

.   .   .

We can do this at home in our bedrooms. Not only do lovers boost each other's testosterone, a woman receives two natural estrogens through sperm. So the big "O" is actually Mother Nature's way to boost these hormones in both men and women. For the act of being open to potentially creating another human life, nature wants to tend the brains of the possible parents and caretakers of that next generation! *This is a new way of looking at making love.* Connecting the dots of science points to this perception. Nature wants us to have pleasure from making love. The better the lovemaking, the bigger the pay off. Intimacy takes care of our brains and thus the entire family and the kiddos to come.

I love that scene in *The First Wives Club* where Goldie Hawn sits back in a plastic surgeon's chair and demands, "Fill 'er up." She is referring to getting her lips plumped up with filler. That is what orgasms and hugging and lovemaking can do for your brain and for many other tissues, too.

Estrogen and testosterone are rumbling plate tectonics with enormous overlap. No single hormone is better than the other; they're just different, but both are downright essential in men and women. Great sex keeps downloading more hormones into our tissues and brain so we can keep upgrading ourselves.

Now that you have the background, let's delve into the similarities and differences between Venus and Mars that need to be embraced for you to really and truly enjoy your mutual embraces.

CHAPTER 2

Venus & Mars Give and Take

*G*abriella was married to Chris, an older but sexy man. Chris was on testosterone replacement and enjoying a high sex drive even though he was in his mid-seventies. *Gabriella hoped to keep up with Chris, who had merely gone to a local Low T hormone center, been tested and treated, and was friskier right out of the chute. (The term "low T" describes a man with low blood levels of testosterone.)*

Gabriella went to a women's hormone medical center. She was put through more rigorous testing, with higher costs and intricate recommendations. It took a full six months for the docs to figure out the most optimal dosages for her. She did get a higher sex drive, more enjoyment out of intimacy, and a huge improved sense of well-being, but she had to jump through a lot of hoops to pull this off. Chris, in contrast, got them fast and easily with less muss and fuss.

Why? Women are more complex. Men, you may wish she was simpler, lower maintenance, and drama-free, but that ain't the way Mother Nature arranged things.

Men and women have the same hormones

Men and women have the exact same hormones, *but in different amounts*. For example, women have five to ten percent of the amount of testosterone that men have. This translates into women naturally making about .3 mg of testosterone daily compared to a typical male making about 7 grams, or ten times as much. Of great interest is the research that suggests that *women are more sensitive and responsive to testosterone* signaling than men are, so that a small amount inside the female body goes a very long way. As far as hormones go, parts per million, billion, and even trillion make enormous differences.

Men have relatively less estrogen than women when they are younger, but if they age in an *unhealthy* manner—getting heavier and out of shape with less muscle mass and more fat cells, or drinking to excess, which boosts excessive estrogen production—then their estrogen levels rise while their testosterone levels fall. It's more difficult for men to stay manly, sexy, and interested if they have inside them more Venus than Mars. Men need estrogen. But not too much. Hormones demand Goldilocks "just right" balance. If a man's estrogen levels are too high or out of balance with his testosterone levels, the bonk level in the bedroom won't register on the Richter scale.

. . .

*Men continue to be simpler and
women more complex.*

. . .

At the receptor level

Men continue to be simpler and women more complex. Remember, receptors are satellites dishes that catch the hormone signals that tell cells how to run your body and life. Receptors, their number per cell and their actions, continue to reflect this theme of Venus being more complex and Mars more simple. The human body has *many more* estrogen receptors than testosterone receptors. And the actions of these

12

estrogen receptors are much more *diverse* when compared to what happens once a male receptor is signaled.

Difference in numbers:

- There are 20,000 to 50,000 estrogen receptors per normal healthy cells that are designed to receive estrogen email.

- There are 10,000 to 20,000 male receptors per healthy normal cells that take signals from testosterone.

Since there are many (up to sixty) estrogen-acting hormone molecules, there are many estrogen receptors—estrogen receptor alpha, estrogen receptor beta, estrogen receptor gamma, delta, receptor X, and a number of others—and still more being discovered all the time. Each receptor, upon receiving an estrogen email, delivers *different* messages to the cell.

In comparison, testosterone has only *two* main receptors, alpha and beta, which do basically similar things. PS: There happens to be another testosterone receptor, mainly in the heart, called *beta-1 adrenergic,* but it is not considered a basic testosterone receptor.

When estrogen receptors receive an email, their actions are vastly varied compared to testosterone receptors.

- When estrogen delivers its message to the *alpha*-receptor, it *stimulates growth.*

- When estrogen delivers its message to the *beta*-receptor, its signals *controlled growth.*

These are two very different actions. They are almost opposite actions.

Why would this be, that estrogen delivers such black-and-white signals? Because nature is all about balance and safety. Nature designed one estrogen signal to stimulate growth. Estrogen makes your heart thump, your gut squeeze, and your mind think. These are powerful growth signals. But then nature provided a powerful built-in control, a fail-safe, so estrogen won't promote growth *out of control.* Thus, estrogen can deliver signals of *growth,* as well as signals of *controlled growth.* That's nature—an equal opportunity employer.

Estradiol is the most well-known and straightforward estrogen; compared to other estrogens, it delivers the most balanced message. Why? Estradiol delivers half its emails to estrogen receptor alpha and half its emails to estrogen receptor beta. Balance.

Testosterone has only two receptors, and they have less diverse actions. Testosterone is not such a growth promoter as estrogen and it doesn't need the same growth control. And as you've learned, it's a younger hormone on the planet in evolutionary speak. So it didn't have as much time as it evolved to need as many checks and balances.

No right or wrong, just different.

Also, the main testosterone receptor is more similar to the progesterone receptor (the other major female hormone) than it is to the estrogen receptor. In fact, all the other sex steroids are more similar to each other than to estrogen.

Once again, estrogen stands alone, more complex than all the other receptors. And all the other hormones. So that woman in front of you, at her deepest biology, is set up to be *unstoppably complex.*

Blood levels of estrogen and testosterone

Testosterone is made and squirted into the bloodstream at a fairly constant level day in and day out. It is slightly higher in the morning, and some studies say that it rises a bit on weekends exclusively in men (when men can go home, relax, and turn their focus away from work). But moment to moment, most of the time, testosterone levels in the blood can be called "Steady Freddy."

In comparison, estrogen levels erratically go up and down, "Seesaw Sally."

Estrogen blood levels have high peaks at least twice in a month (at ovulation and before menses). They go very high *up* and then very low *down* (with, of course, some variation from woman to woman). In fact, when estrogen replacement is given to mature women, it is often prescribed for so many days "on" cycled with a few days "off" (called a *hormone holiday*) to mimic the natural ebb and flow, up and down, of estrogen in the bodies of younger women. The more you mimic Mother Nature, the less trouble you get in.

The take-home is that women's estrogen levels rise and then fall substantially at various times of the month. If you look at a graph of estrogen, you will see that its levels are all over the map every 30 days. This means that at the hormonal level, her biologic wiring, a woman is set up to be an *emotional tornado.*

When men or women are given testosterone replacement, they can take it daily. It doesn't need any cycling, as it doesn't naturally go up and down in either the male or female body. It does not have striking highs or lows; it is not all over the place. A man is set up to be more solid than a woman.

To summarize how hormones are set up by nature:

- Estrogen is more complicated than testosterone; testosterone is simpler.

- Estrogen includes 60 versions of estrogenic molecules with three major estrogens; testosterone is one major molecule with five versions of itself.

- Estrogen has more receptors per cell; testosterone has less.

- Estrogen has more diverse receptors with diverse actions; testosterone has less receptors with less diverse actions.

- Estrogen is the oldest hormone on the planet—the "cougar" hormone.

- Testosterone acts rocklike, steady, like a Zen hormone; estrogens are naturally more up and down and emotional.

Venus and Mars

These differences between estrogen and testosterone explain why it is so difficult for men and women to understand each other.

Men can sit and think of "one thing" or "nothing" for hours, while women can have sixty thoughts flying through their brains within minutes. Men are clearly wired for more simplicity and silence. And women for more complication and sound.

Honoring these differences will help to deepen and harmonize your intimacies.

. . .

Hormones are powerful hard-wired signaling molecules inside our physiologies.

. . .

Hormones are powerful hard-wired signaling molecules inside our physiologies. Women are wired like their female hormones—convoluted, diverse, and erratic. Some women are upset that I make estrogen sound more emotional than testosterone. They worry that this contributes to women being regarded as "less" than men. But at the molecular level, women *are* set up to be more emotional. This does not prevent millions of women from being levelheaded and stable and developing successful skills.

The point is that the molecules act this way, and there is a deep molecular reverberation that plays a role in the female life experience.

Mother Nature is all about the next generation. I believe that keeping women emotional, heightened in awareness, "all over the place," and responsive to multiple cues in the environment makes women more likely to hear the baby if it gets into danger. Women are wide open to be able to hear and take care of the next generation.

The Hormone Love Language

To ask a woman to be feminine and sexy, but then also to ask her to be "solid and steady" the way a man is wired, is asking her to go against her hormonal template and physiology. It's asking her to go against her hard-wired hormone inner language. It doesn't mean that she is Velcroed to *reactivity* and can't be anything but emotional, but it means that this rhythm, tendency, or "default" is deeply rooted in her molecular nooks and crannies, and she inevitably bumps into it, especially when backed into emotional or fearful corners. *Men, get this!*

Also, for a woman to want a man to be her safe harbor, her steadfast hero, but then ask him to be with her on her emotional roller coaster or to empathize like her girlfriends do, goes against his physiology. This doesn't mean that men shouldn't strive to develop empathy, kindness, and generosity, but it explains basic tendencies and differences. *Ladies, get this!*

In response to the feminine movement, many men seem to have abdicated their masculinity in an attempt to be more politically correct. But it isn't working! It isn't honoring how men and women have been hard-wired deep at the atomic level of their molecules.

Men. When a woman asks you where you are going to dinner that night, today it is not uncommon to get a response like, "Wherever you want." Or when woman supplies a phone number on a dating site to have a man call, the man often responds, "You call me whenever you can," or "Here's my number, you call me." In other words, men who are not sure what it means to be a man today are taking the back seat. They think they are being more politically correct, but they are being more feminine, not male-like. This lack of assertiveness does not make a woman move closer to you. It pushes her away. *Men, get this!*

Nature intended women's physiology to be more all over the place (more emotional), to be a better mom, and to see all and be all to the family. This up-and-down, hard-wired tendency needs you, the man, to be a rock. Take charge. Don't say, "Wherever you want to go." Instead let her know, "I have planned for us to go here." Or, "I am taking you there." These type of sentences are manly. They are steady. They are how you are hard-wired. This type of language lets a woman know, even in this small way, that you want to take care of her. This language makes a woman feel more secure with you, deep inside, even if she doesn't realize why or have the words to say it herself.

Men, get this! Be strong. Your molecules long for you to take back your maleness. You can do so without being a chauvinist.

Women, get this! Let the man take some of his power back; in this way you will be honoring his molecules. Support him to be the Rock of Gibraltar you really long for.

True story. A number of years ago, the hormone think tank I was part of at Tulane University was sponsoring a conference where the most high-ly-respected scientists in hormone research were sharing their newest data. A meet-and-greet party was held the first night at a high-rise in downtown New Orleans. I was finally going to meet , face to face in a smaller friendlier setting, so many of the famous scientists whose papers I had been devouring for years.

Within minutes, a small group of around ten scientists had gathered around the drink and food table—all women. We looked out over the twinkling city lights, munching, drinking, and talking. Being in awe, I stood back to listen. I was sure I would hear something scientifically earth-shaking, but within minutes, as often happens when women gather, the talk turned toward men.

What was said amazed me. These high-powered but kind and friendly women disclosed how displeased they were with their long-term hus-bands. One woman had been married for thirty years and was happy. But the rest were debating whether divorcing was better than staying and compromising.

Why were they unhappy? They pretty much all agreed that their men were good guys, good providers, and good friends, but there was no true romantic love. These women felt true love had passed them by. None of them had great intimacy, which to my amazement they shared openly. None of them felt that their men were the love of their lives. These women were strong, but at home they missed being treated as

women. They missed strong men. Today's male and female dance partners are tripping all over each other's feet.

At a recent book club meeting in Austin, all thirty women started
discussing their marriages. Only two women were happy with their
long-term husbands. The other twenty-eight were longing for love.
They wanted great romance, intimacy, and communication. They wanted to feel like feminine women to masculine men. They mainly felt
overworked, misunderstood, and too pooped to make love. When they
"did it," what they got wasn't worth it. But since leaving doesn't guar-
antee finding what you want, they were debating the compromise of
staying with what they already had.

Many patients in my office admit they are in the same situation.

Today's roles are mixed up. We've lost our maleness and femaleness
based on how we are set up by nature at our most hormonal and molecular levels. Intimacy is faltering. Deep inside too many relationships,
Mars and Venus wonder if there isn't something better out there. But
the truth is, when you translate the hormone language of love into communication inside and outside the bedroom, you can get back your
male and female satisfaction.

Awakened love and sex, which is what nature meant you to have, high
in pleasure and brain and relationship-boosting benefits, can save the
relationship you are in or the one you are dreaming about.

Testosterone is less about bonding and more about physical (not emotional) grounding. Studies have consistently shown that testosterone
levels go down a bit in prospective fathers and men with children compared to male adults without children or who are not married. This
lowering of testosterone when having a wife or child has been regarded
by researchers as Mother Nature making men better family members,
more able to bond with their children, and less likely to leave the
household to go after other women. Mix this with the estrogenic influx
from today's chemical toxic world (which we will learn about soon),
junk food diets, and mixed-up relationship roles, it is easy for a guy to
become feminized. So one must look to testing hormones and hormone

replacement if necessary. And to consider behaviors that honor the sex hormone molecules.

In men with higher levels of blood testosterone, their physiology drives their desire toward sex on a more physical basis, and emotions do not need to enter into the picture as much as they do naturally with women. So ladies, if you want your man to be manly, realize that within a relationship he is not just another girlfriend, one who pays the bills. Get this!

Once we realize how hardwired these differences are in men and women, we can choose to not *overreact* or consistently *personalize* the differences when they show up. And to behave in ways that allow our own molecules and those of our mates to be in harmony and connection. I believe this bigger picture of Mars and Venus will lead to more appreciation, acceptance, peace, and ultimately, more mind-boggling sex.

At the atomic level: the "H-bomb"

A critical difference in comparing estrogen and testosterone occurs at the level of the atom. This is the first time, I believe, that this specific comparison has been discussed in print.

Atoms are the building blocks of molecules. Molecules are made up of atoms held together by chemical bonds. The most critical divergence between men and women is the difference of only *one atom*, the *hydrogen atom*, which I have dubbed the "H-bomb." Here's the story.

While I was writing *Safe Hormones, Smart Women* (a book demonstrating the evidence-based science behind the safety and benefits of bioidentical hormone replacement), I was a scholar at an estrogen-driven think tank at Tulane University. I was privileged to work with the absolute top researchers and academicians in the world of hormones, such as the scientists who discovered estrogen receptors alpha and beta.

I had an out-of-the-box idea. Tom Bishop PhD. was one of the first investigators to create theoretical molecular modeling of estrogen molecules and knew the ins and outs of estrogen molecules better than most humans on the planet. I took the risk and called Dr. Bishop at his home. I asked if he would consider spending a number of hours literally sitting and staring at both the estrogen and testosterone molecules. Maybe he would see something new lurking at the molecular/atomic levels that had never been observed before.

Dr. Bishop was unenthusiastic. I wasn't offering thousands of grant dollars, although I wanted to pay him something. Finally he said, "I just can't imagine finding anything that hasn't been reported before." But I was determined and eventually we agreed that he would sit and stare at both molecules and I would pay for a $300 bottle of wine his wife wanted for her birthday. We both laughed and hung up.

A few months went by. I left messages but didn't hear back. Darn. I thought he blew the odd request off.

Then, a week after my book went to press (too late to add any new information), I got a call from Dr. Bishop, who said, "You know, Lindsey, when you first asked me to do this, I honestly thought you were crazy. But you were going to pay for that overpriced bottle of wine, so I did sit down, feeling foolish, and stared dutifully at those molecules. After about two hours, what I saw made the hair on the back of my neck stand up."

Dr. Bishop had seen a very basic difference between estradiol and testosterone, and what he saw, to his knowledge, no other scientist or doctor had ever seen before or written about.

The testosterone and estrogen molecules are almost exactly the same. The male molecule is slightly bigger, but not by much, and they have exactly the same benzene rings (the inner ring-like structure the atoms hang on). But Tom saw an astronomic difference.

He said, "When I saw this, I couldn't believe it. I am not sure what to make of it, like in relating to larger systems such as personality or how men and women are spoken about in religious terms, but this is real. At the atomic level, *testosterone can only take and estrogen can only give.*"

His wife got that bottle of wine.

This is what he saw: At the molecular level, testosterone has an empty space where estrogen can donate a hydrogen atom, or some other molecule can donate there. Estrogen, on the other hand, has an extra hydrogen atom, and compared to testosterone, estrogen can only give it away. It has no space available to take in another hydrogen atom.

So at the very basic structure of the male and female hormones, the male hormone is set up to "take" and the female hormone is set up to "give."

Testosterone

Estrogen

See the lower left corner of each molecule? On the far left, testosterone has an oxygen atom (O) but is missing a hydrogen atom (H), and has room to add one on. Estrogen has both (HO) and can only give that hydrogen atom away.

But the story continues

I sent this above part of the book to my mentor John McLachlan, the internationally recognized estrogen expert who headed the estrogen think tank I was part of at Tulane University.

John immediately wrote back, "Linds, I think you ought to run this viewpoint by Dr. Michael E. Baker. He's the top-of-the-heap estrogen dude. Michael understands estrogen nuances better than anyone else. I copied him on your and Tom's thoughts."

So Dr. Michael E. Baker, a professor and scientist at University of California at Davis, and I began a flurry of voluminous email exchanges.

Dr. Baker said, "Devaki, you are the second person to ever ask me this question." Dr. Baker was, in fact, writing new papers about these estrogen/testosterone shades of gray at the very moment John put us in touch. In Dr. Baker's research, he'd spent hundreds of hours looking at both estrogen and testosterone. How they are alike. How they are not. And no one was blackmailing him with fine wine for his wife!

• • •

At the atomic level testosterone can only give and estrogen can give and take.

• • •

The molecules show that testosterone can only take, as Dr. Bishop noted. But Dr. Baker felt a strong case could be made that estrogen herself can both give and take. Dr. Baker sent me multiple molecular diagrams in which he printed arrows showing that, yes, estrogen freely gives, but she can take, too. But Dr. Baker agreed that testosterone is only a taker!

It seems that whether estrogen only gives, or gives and takes, Mother Nature lubed the gears of testosterone to be set up and ready to RECEIVE!

Translated into sex

What do the above scientific viewpoints mean in the bedroom and in relationships? Women are biologically intricate. They are used to speaking and listening much longer than male molecules. They are older, more complex, and more giving.

So any man wanting to woo and win a woman needs to approach her on *complex* levels. You've got to talk to her a bit, touch her a bit, laugh and listen and play a bit, hug a bit, and then go for the gusto. (*This doesn't mean you can never go fast and furious and have a good time, but in general, women respond best to appetizers before the main meal.*)

Women take real note of your facial expressions. They listen to your words and don't forget. They long for your touch and hugs. Cuddling is very meaningful to women. They want to give, but women want to know that you appreciate what they are giving. They are set up to give and to respond to attention on a variety of levels. They are not wired for "wham, bam, thank you ma'am" or sex without intentional touch, supportive words, and some wooing.

But women, on the other hand, need to realize that men love to be given to! To be looked up to. To feel respected. To be honored. To receive.

Men are very responsive to women who show and give them admiration, attention, and loyalty. Women, you can gift men adoring words, ask how they might like to be given to, even ask what you might do to help set up the romantic mood. Also, letting men know they pleasure you can be a gift back to them.

Men love when a woman receives pleasure and then lets her partner know exactly how much pleasure he has given her. How? With words, or moans, or movement. Respond. The more you respond and he can hear it, feel it, and get it, the more you are actually giving. Giving the gift of pleasure right back to him, letting him see and hear how his giving affects you—this is "mutuality of biology" in action. Both your brains and hormones should be humming and shimmying in harmony.

CHAPTER 3

Male and Female Hardwired

*L*ayla and Larry were at odds with each other. They were high school sweethearts but now in their early 20's something was very wrong. Their forward-thinking psychologist had graduated them from couple's therapy, saying she thought they now needed hormonal therapy. They had lived together for four years and had been contemplating marriage, but Larry was on the edge of bolting. He was fed up with how emotional and scattered Layla could be.

They had a lot of positives going for them: great sex, good conversation, they treated each other's families kindly, and both loved golf and Scrabble. But Layla (even though she was a trainer with a buffed body) could go from calm to screaming in 30 seconds. It could take her weeks (if ever) to let go of any argument.

We tested Layla's hormones. Progesterone calms the brain. Her levels were so low they were beneath the detection capabilities of the laboratory. Even though she was young, replacing progesterone gave Layla a steadier and happier personality. Larry, learning that women are set up by nature to be more reactive than males, stopped pressuring her to act otherwise. This also contributed to her deeper peace.

On the other hand, Layla learned that Larry, being less reactive and less communicative, was simply being manly. She stopped yelling at him to get him to talk. She focused more on his actions than his words. She stopped expecting him to act like a girlfriend.

Within three months they decided to get married and invited me to the wedding.

All brains are not created equal

While both men and women use their brains to think and carry out similar functions, there are major differences in the ways their brains are structured. Translating these differences into the bedroom can go a long way in improving how you and your partner get along, communicate, and work out issues, as well as how you both can experience earth-shattering sex.

With neuroimaging technology, we can look inside the brains of men and women and directly see the gender differences. On average, men have larger brains than women; this difference begins to occur at four or five years of age. However, just as some women are larger than some men, some women have larger brains than some men. It's variable.

Men, whatever you do, do not conclude that men are *smarter* than women because the male brains are generally bigger. Consider that, on average, a whale's brain is about 20 times larger than a human's brain, or that birds in the corvid family (crows, jays, ravens, etc.), with their smaller bird brains, have been shown to be just as smart as chimps and gorillas!

Women are more right-brained

It has been clearly demonstrated that women have thicker outer brain layers (cortices) at two specific areas on the *right* side of their brain— the *inferior parietal* and *posterior temporal* regions. These two areas in women's brains are on average 0.45 mm thicker than these same regions in male brains. In brain terrain terms, this is substantial. It's accurate to say that women are more *right-brained* compared to men, and magnetic resonance imaging has confirmed it.

The inferior parietal area is involved in the perception of *emotions*, from facial expressions and other sensory information to language and body image. The posterior temporal region focuses on *word* processing. So women are wired to have more emotions and use more words: their gray matter makes them do it.

. . .

Female brains are constructed for empathy and communicating with others, but also for worrying.

. . .

Female brains are constructed for *empathy* and *communicating* with others, but also for *worrying*, including worry about body image and how they look. Her brain responds to what you show on your face and to all the words you say. She very much cares about how you see her and how you make her feel about how she sees herself. If she asks you if her bottom looks too large in a pair of jeans, tread very carefully in your reply. Her brain will take it very seriously, she won't forget, and she'll go over and over these words in her head, and probably with all her girlfriends.

Translated into sex

Because body image is a highly developed part of women's brains, men need to show women how attractive they are by authentic expressions of admiration and arousal as they look at their bodies. Because words are important to women, men should use words generously, along with touch, for showing their admiration and when making love.

Because women's brains are more attentive to emotions and facial expressions, look interested, show approval, and at least say something you like about her body. This goes a long way to nudge her brain into liking you and enjoying sex with you. To make love with a woman and not compliment one thing about her body will greatly lower her enjoyment of sex with you.

Female brains and language skills

Brains have speech areas. Two of these areas are called the Wernicke and the Broca language-associated regions. These brain areas are much larger in the female brain, from 17 to almost 30% larger. Yikes!

This creates a lot of room for misunderstanding between men and women. This research showing that size matters was first published by scientists at the School of Communication Disorders, University of Sydney, Australia in 1997, so we have known this for a while. But have you? Larger anatomical brain areas in women translate to superior language skills. Her brain makes her talk a lot, often in that annoying way (at least to men).

. . .

The hippocampus, the brain area of memory, is larger in wormen. This is antoher reason women don't forget.

. . .

The hippocampus, the brain area of memory, is larger in women. This is another reason women don't forget. By the way, meditation has been found to boost hippocampal size and memory in both males and females. Sit together in peace and quiet. Hold hands and breathe together for three silent breaths. *Silent hand holding and breathing in sync can reboot relationship glitches.*

Men are often in awe that women remember every word they utter. That they can talk so much. And so fast. Women's brains are anatomically crafted for a greater propensity to speak faster, to remember, and to experience emotions. And to worry if their butt is assuming the shape of their favorite chair.

Translated into sex

Ladies, when you see him start to get overwhelmed with what you are saying, back off. Don't continue drowning his smaller anatomical brain regions in words that comfort you but not him. (Boy, I wish I had known this in my last relationship!)

Men, are her words too much for you? Kiss her gently to quiet her. Laugh and remind her to be quiet. Laugh together. Touch more. Be her rock. Hold her. When you cuddle, her testosterone starts to rise and this grounds her. She is wired, remember, to respond exquisitely to testosterone and maleness.

Men, when you are speaking to women, don't say things you can't back up down the road, because she will never let you hear the end of it. Say your truth. Don't hide it under shallow words that will come back later to haunt you. Express your truth kindly and gently, not abruptly or in a rude tone; she won't forget that either. Avoid silence. That feels okay to you but it actually hurts her. *Default to touching and holding.* This calms her, quiets her, and boosts her testosterone levels. Both your brains will feel better.

Male brains have more activity in spatial areas

Men don't have to ask for directions because spatial sense is more forged into their brains. This advantage for spatial abilities (the ability to mentally rotate two- and three-dimensional objects) has been widely documented in men. This means they are keen observers of the shape of things—especially women. Shapely women, or women they appreciate as shapely, turn men on; *his brain makes it happen.*

Translated into sex

Ladies, if you want to keep your men interested, take care of yourself, feel good in your body suit, comfy with who you are, and present yourself in ways that enhance your attractiveness to the men you care about.

You don't have to have a perfect figure by any means, but if you feel comfortable inside yourself, if you feel sexy and attractive and exude sexiness, if you lean back and strike a pose that you know shows off your best features or your sensuous side, this turns men on. If you are unsure of yourself, uncomfortable in how you feel about how you look, feel out of shape and unattractive, this turns men off (and you both lose out). It's not diabolical or unfair or men being mean; male brain structure makes males see women in this shape-oriented way.

· · ·

It's not diabolical or unfair or men being mean;
male brain structure makes males see women
in this shape-oriented way.

· · ·

To keep your man happy, get more comfortable in your own skin, smell nice,
be clean, and turn on your man's brain!

Smell is the one cranial nerve, the one brain input, that cannot be turned off. It is always on. Thus, many of us are deeply influenced romantically by the scent of those we attempt to mate with, even if we are not aware that any of this is happening.

There is remarkable size and diversity to your scent organs. They contain a huge number of receptors and genes, more than any other sense. Perceiving scents relies heavily on the "very first event." The first time you smell someone, that scent "stays" with you. The main organ of smell, the olfactory bulb, is extremely sensitive to scents, even ones below your awareness level. For example, if you consume a lot of processed foods and meats, even though you do not recognize how your genitalia and body give off a scent, they do give off a different scent than someone who is eating more *cleanly.*

A diet excessively high in poor fatty food choices blunts the sensitivity of smelling scents! You may smell less desirable and you can't even detect it. But the more you eat a healthy diet, with fish, seeds, nuts, and other good fats like avocado and coconut, the better you continue to give off scent and to also perceive it in others.

Sulfur-containing foods, like garlic, have been shown to make men smell more romantically attractive to women from their underarm areas!

On your first date, take a shower, use essential oils, and be thoroughly clean to make sure your scent is siren-like to the one you hope to connect with.

The scent of romance

In younger women, hormones help their bodies produce molecules of attraction called *pheromones*. Pheromones release subliminal scents that make these women appealing to men. Pheromonal production is stimulated by estrogens. And estrogens also stimulate the sense of smell so that these younger, higher estrogen-containing women, can better smell male pheromones (men give off scents, too). So younger women give off sensual, romantic scents and they are also very good at perceiving sensual scents in males.

. . .

Studies run on animals suggest that hormone therapies can reboot the ability to give off and perceive pheromones.

. . .

Menopausal women have less estrogen. Some younger women these days—with our toxic environment, poor diets, and sustained stress—are also making less estrogen. When estrogen blood levels tank, pheromones tank, too. So women give off less attraction molecules, and they perceive male scent less well. Remember, estrogen is a major factor enabling the ability of smelling. Thus the external toxic environment may be dinging desire in young women this way. Also, if a maturing woman is not on hormone therapy, she gives off less pheromones and perceives less pheromones. This may contribute to the lack of desire as women age.

Studies run on animals suggest that hormone therapies can reboot the ability to give off and perceive pheromones. Human studies run on commercial pheromonal formulas have shown them to be effective in terms of desiring more touch, cuddling, and connection.

Males exude subliminal scents of attraction, too. So men also need to eat well and be conscious of smelling attractive. But not everyone has equal sensitivity to scents. It's individual. I know most of my life I seem to have been run by my nose, but this certainly is not the case for everyone. Remember, much of this romantic scent interchange is happening below your conscious awareness. This means you are not always aware that these scent influences are going on. But it makes sense that keeping yourself smelling good, consuming a healthy diet, or testing and replacing hormones if necessary so that your body emanates pleasing scents is part of a larger picture of attraction.

Men and Women Since Time Began

From the beginning of time, men and women have been intertwined. This is an astounding story that very few scientists and physicians know about yet, since it's brand new at the time of writing this book.

First, a small reminder. If you recall, a hormone is a two-part proposition. You first have to have a receptor that acts as a satellite dish to receive a hormonal message. Secondly, you have to have a signaling hormone that sends that message. If you have a receptor but no hormone, no signal can be sent.

Where do the signals go? The receptor takes the signals and passes them forward. They are delivered to genes deep inside cells to tell the cells what to do. Without these signals, the internal computer of your body freezes and you feel tired, dumb, and certainly not sexy.

According to Dr. Michael E. Baker, the world's top authority on estrogen's evolution, in the beginning there were only estrogen receptors.

The testosterone receptor did not yet exist! And neither did the main estrogen, estradiol. First on the scene was the lonely estrogen receptor waiting to receive an email so she could *talk* to genes.

This was occurring in early primitive vertebrates (vertebrates have backbones). For you geeks out there, this was in "animals" called amphioxus, which are a close ancestor of lampreys (the jawless fish). This early life contained the first estrogen receptors.

So who signaled the first estrogen receptor? Remember, there was not yet any estrogen hormone, only an estrogen receptor. Who first came knocking at that estrogen receptor's door?

Dr. Baker has been pondering this question for years. He said there were several signals that first delivered messages to the estrogen receptor. One was an early *male-like* molecule. It was only male-like as it didn't yet have its own male receptor, so it couldn't be an actual male hormone. This male molecule (called *Adiol*) signaled the first estrogen receptors.

Thus a male molecule first *nudged* estrogen receptors to send the first estrogen signals. Sort of like giving her a male molecular "rib" to help estrogen go forth and be all that she could be.

If today the original estrogen stood up in front of a microphone at the Academy Awards, she'd probably be saying, "I am only here tonight because of all that *maleness* has done for me."

. . .

At the most archival level of life, there has always been an energetic resonance of maleness and femaleness needing each other.

. . .

In the beginning, the first female signal needed male help to deliver that signal. At the most archival level of life, there has always been an energetic resonance of *maleness* and *femaleness* needing each other.

Dr. Baker says there was yet another substance that helped the earliest estrogen signals be delivered. What was that? Fat! In the form of cholesterol. So the first estrogen was able to deliver hormonal signals because of *fat*. Ask any woman and I'm sure she'd say, "I could have told you that!"

Mars and Venus (and fat) have been molecularly hugging and enmeshing since the earliest life forms.

Dr. Baker said that some time after estrogen receptors got used to receiving signals, estradiol, the most well-recognized estrogen, began to be made. Thus estradiol became and has continued to be the most basic signal for estrogen receptors. It would be some time before the male receptor came to exist and be part of the evolving body's signaling system.

Thus, only estrogen could first, in essence, *speak*. She did this for millions of years before any other hormone could signal. So *speaking* is unfathomably hardwired into the estrogen lineage. *Guys, get this!*

. . .

*For millions of years the male signal
didn't have a voice.*

. . .

For millions of years the male signal didn't have a voice. It helped estrogen have hers but didn't have its own. Is this why many women complain that men seem more insecure in the communication realm than in the physical? Also, maleness and femaleness, looking at each hormone's historical relationship and present day atomic one, are confusing. At the level of the atoms, testosterone can only take. But for eons testosterone's job description was to *give*. Thus, nature has set up an on-going challenge between males and females since time began. We need each other but are hard-wired with contrasting differences. Frustrations are built-in. Understanding this helps you not take conflict so personally and enjoy the friction. If you think true love means happily ever after without challenge, you are not realizing that nature longs for us to grow. By growing from efforts to accept each other's differences with a chilled-out attitude, we earn ecstasy. Understanding all this helps us achieve peace and success within love.

Dr. Baker also wrote in yet another one of our many emails, "Well, as I have commented in a couple of seminars, the estrogen (female) receptor evolved before the androgen (male) receptor. Thus, we could also say that Adam could be regarded as having been made from Eve's rib.

Apparently the rib story can go either way.

Ultimately, estrogen had the first receptor no matter who sent the message to that receptor. *She's* used to speaking her own mind as she was the only one on the signaling block for over 400 million years doing just that. But yes, she needed help.

Why would nature have a male hormone signal the first estrogen receptor? I asked this to Dr. Baker. His answer made me laugh. Dr. Baker said that the male hormone was much easier to make as it was much less complex! (And he hadn't read my book yet.) Dr. Baker said it took a while for Mother Nature to create estradiol, as that process was much more multifaceted.

Whatever the exact story, nature has consistent themes. The feminine evolved first and is more involved. Gender bending has been going on forever. And, yes, we have always needed one another; there is absolutely no evolutionary doubt about that!

Men and women, as the gender stories continue, also have deep-rooted *dissimilarities* in their gray matter that can make these intermeshings ever so frustrating.

Let's now take a look at these differences in the brain.

Venus and Mars gray matter gender-benders

The male and female brains are hardwired somewhat differently. Once you understand these dissimilarities—that are deeply rooted and that we all bring to the table when attempting to love someone, you can gently laugh at what shows up rather than pull your proverbial hair out.

- Female babies produce more estrogen, and have more verbal and emotional brain circuitry right from the get-go.

- Brain cells feminized by estrogen promote genes that encourage faster brain development. This continues through puberty, during which time girl brains develop about two years earlier than boy brains.

- As adults, women have 11 percent more neurons than men in the brain centers for speaking and *listening*. Their brain is wired to hear more than the male brain.

- Male babies have higher levels of testosterone that potentially tamp down verbal and emotional circuitry. Hear that? That means lower listening and talking skills!

- Female babies immediately begin studying faces more intently than male babies, which further shapes their brain development and encourages more empathy, communication, gut feelings, emotional memory, and anger control.

- The emotion-processing center of the brain, the *amygdala*, reaches its full development about one-and-a-half years *earlier* in the female than the male. The amygdala plays an important role in the responses of fear and courage as well as certain types of memory.

- Women's brains are built to forget fewer details than men's brains.

- Men are more about focusing on what's in front of them. They can easily focus on only one thing or on nothing at all.

- Women's brains are more about focusing on everything. Face it, women just have more stressful brains!

The ebb and flow of female hormones

Levels of estrogen and progesterone, the two major female hormones, cycle *up* and *down* throughout a female's adult life, making women more prone to *ups* and *downs* in mood and at much greater risk of depression and anxiety compared to men. This ebb and flow also creates a greater focus on relationships, nesting, and love, which create a sense of stability to calm all this up and down motion. *The female physiology longs for stability.*

. . .

The female physiology longs for stability.

. . .

Males secrete stable levels of testosterone throughout most of each month and year, which makes them less prone to depression, more solid and stable, and *not as focused on relationships and nesting* as women.

Male and female reactions to stress

During any stressful event, women secrete more stress hormones (such as *cortisol*, the flight-or-fight hormone). Adrenocorticotropic hormone (ACTH) is made in the brain to turn on the release of the stress hormone, cortisol, from the adrenal glands. Compared to men, ACTH blood levels are higher at all ages in all women. So the female brain is wired to be very reactive to stress. And once females release stress hormones, these hormone levels remain elevated for longer periods of time compared to men.

. . .

During any stressful event, women secrete more stress hormones.

. . .

You two can argue at breakfast and his stress hormones are back down to normal before he gets into the car to drive off to work, while yours may stay elevated for the next several weeks. Or months!

The reason for this difference may be that stress hormones heighten our awareness. Women are wired to be more wide open to the environment in case there is danger to the baby (even when there is no baby).

Men also secrete stress hormones, like cortisol, when under stress. There is some evidence that high levels of cortisol can tamp down testosterone blood levels and consequently lower men's sex drive. Perhaps nature created this temporary reduction of testosterone so that men could focus on what they need to do to increase their chance of survival, and that of their family, in an emergency. But male cortisol levels go back down to normal much faster than they do in women.

. . .

But male cortisol levels go back down to normal
much faster than they do in women.

. . .

The levels in women may take days, weeks, months, or may still be high from an event that took place several years ago. I kid you not. Her female brain and how it is hard-wired (especially exposure to severe stress during her first four years of life) make her do it.

Translated into sex

These are gender-specific physiologic realities, the real behavior reality show that actually directs our actions. The higher levels of stress hormones and their longer duration of secretion, cause women to be more easily stressed out, and for much longer than seems to make sense, at least to their male mate. The interactions between testosterone and stress may take a toll on men's sexual desire, but usually not for long.

So guys, don't get so angry when she gets upset or stays upset; her biology makes her do it. And women, don't expect your man to be full of desire for you when he's under a lot of stress. Both of you will benefit if you try to lower each other's stress levels or to understand each other's response to what is perceived as stress.

Interestingly, nothing can reduce stress levels like a good tumble in bed with your mate. Sounds like a catch-22, doesn't it? How can you have a good tumble if she's still stressed over an argument you had last week, and his stress caused his testosterone to plummet? The answer is to begin by being aware of each other's stress and understanding the effects of stress on your mate. Then search for ways to relieve it. A glass of wine, soft music, mutual massage, whispered sweet nothings in the ear and a few squirts of oxytocin up the nose (which you will learn about soon). Read Chapter 14 together and you'll find a way.

Falling in love

Women are more likely to fall in love. Men are more likely to fall in lust.

Of course, some men fall deeply in love, and some women lust heartily after their man. The above statement is about as true as "women are likely to be shorter than men." There are always exceptions, but the statements are generally true, as dictated by different biologies and differing amounts of male and female hormones.

Women are more likely to fall in love because their pituitary glands secrete more of a hormone called *oxytocin* (pronounced *ok-si-toh-suhn*) when making love. Oxytocin is called the "bonding hormone" and the "love hormone" because it causes emotional bonding during love-making (and while breastfeeding a baby). Oxytocin actually promotes activity in the brain where *intimate connection* and *empathy* occur. Yes, there is a specific brain region that is all about my favorite vitamin C: connection.

When a woman regularly makes love with her man, the oxytocin in her brain starts to make her "addicted" to him. Her brain wires her to him at a most basic brain level.

41

. . .

*Though men secrete oxytocin as well, they secrete
less of it when making love than women do, so
they do not bond as easily as women do.*

. . .

Though men secrete oxytocin as well, they secrete *less* of it when making love than women do, so they do not bond as easily as women do.
Of course, there is still biochemical individuality and some men secrete
more oxytocin than others. However, the more time couples spend in
eye gazing and actual love-making/bonding sessions, the more oxytocin
both partners secrete. This applies to same-sex partners, too. Some
research suggests that homosexual men are more sensitive to the effects
of oxytocin than heterosexual men, which contributes to who they are
and their abilities of connectivity and emotionality.

But sustained and severe stress can turn off oxytocin's ability to create
empathy and connection. We will talk a lot more about oxytocin in
Chapter 8.

He looks for zing, she looks for safety

Noted anthropologist and love expert Dr. Helen Fisher peered into male
and female brains using fMRIs to see what they look like when they fall
in love. Functional brain MRIs measure brain activity in real-time as a
person responds to stimuli.

She found that for men, the most active regions of the brain are related
to *visual stimuli* and *penile erection*. Men are greatly attracted to good
looks and to women who make them physically responsive and cause
them to get a zing in their penis. In women, regions linked with *emotions* and *memory recall* become active during the mating process, so
women are more attracted to men who seem like they will stick around
and be better providers. Her brain remembers her mother or aunt or

grandmother who told her over and over again that she needs a man that can take good care of her.

Women's brains are made to look for a successful man, and men are set up to look for an attractive woman. A woman doesn't have to be physically beautiful to be attractive to a man as long as she feels attractive and confident. A man doesn't have to be a Fortune 500 rich guy, but he does need to make her feel "safe."

. . .

Happiness is gorgeous.

. . .

Footnote for the ladies: Happiness is gorgeous. When you are happy deep inside, you look much more attractive. A man responds to a woman who is happier, *as if* she is more attractive, because . . . *she is!*

When women experience romantic love, it initiates a mating process to ensure that she has identified a stable man who will stay and take care of her and the baby and not abandon them in times of danger. This is necessary because carrying a child in the womb, nursing it, and paying for it takes a great deal more energy and commitment than producing sperm. It makes sense that classically women have looked toward successful men who seem like substantial providers.

Men are more concerned with a greater degree of attractiveness and physical response. And, biologically speaking, what he needs from a woman, other than sexual arousal and fulfillment, is that she carry his genes into the future (of course, partnership can be a high priority for him, too.) A happy disposition, wide hips and a thin waist, are indicators of health and the ability to bring a healthy child into the world. It makes sense that a great body and a happy persona turn his head.

But emerging research from Northwestern University says that difficult economic times might morph male's brains a bit. Some modern younger men are starting to value *brains over beauty* when choosing long-term mates. Contemporary life has become extremely expensive. While the common view is that our mate choices are evolutionarily "hardwired" in our brains (and therefore minimally responsive to changing) some evolutionary scientists now argue that humans are programmed to be more *flexible* in changing times. This possible new phenomenon is mostly in younger men who worry about affording life in a more expensive world, and hope to have a smart partner to help him pull this off economically. Perhaps it may become a modern version of a dowry.

We need each other

Throughout life there is a win-win, yin-yang relationship between estrogen and testosterone. They go together, like men and women, masculinity and femininity, or penises and vaginas. Nature has designed us to be together, to cooperate with each other, to love each other, to be aroused by each other, to have sex with one another, and to produce and raise children together.

The varying amounts and actions of each hormone make huge differences. That basic atomic H-bomb resonates up through the "give" and "take" of estrogen and testosterone. When you respect these differences, the yin and yang of woman and man fit together well and fulfill each other's needs.

What becomes really interesting is the intertwining of male and female hormones, rather like the intertwining of male and female bodies when making love. Male and female hormones are designed to support and nurture each other in various ways, like the ways that a loving couple ideally support and nurture each other in life.

Here is an example of the intertwining of male and female hormones.

We all need estrogen.

- From the very start of life, this so-called female hormone helps *both* male and female fetuses develop.

- Both genders are exposed to estrogen from their mothers and from estrogen made locally inside their developing brains.

- The amounts and types of early estrogen, the number of estrogen receptors, and other factors help determine the gender of the brain and teach the brain how to use signaling molecules (neurotransmitters) that enable brain (and gut) communication throughout life.

So estrogen is as important to males as to females. Here's an example of how testosterone returns the favor and benefits females.

- Testosterone in the body is broken down into a metabolite called DHT, which is further broken down into another metabolite nicknamed 3B-Adiol, which protects the female breast against breast cancer. (P.S., it also protects prostate cells from turning cancerous, so 3B-Adiol can be a woman's man or a man's man type of hormone helper).

- When a woman becomes deficient in the male hormone testosterone, she can become more vulnerable not only to breast cancer but also to other health woes, including bone loss, muscle wasting, low energy, depression, feelings of anxiety, panic attacks, and feeling overwhelmed.

- Both males and females make estrogen out of male hormones.

- Here's the kicker: a woman with low-T can have a flat-lined sex drive!

What does all this say to those of us who are trying to date and mate with each other? It tells us to *honor the differences* to make love stay.

Nature has designed us to be different, yet to come together, to support and nurture each other, to fit into each other's bodies and each other's minds. As the French say with enthusiasm, *vive la différence!*

And as my grandmother used to say, "*The heck with them if they can't appreciate the difference between an apricot and a banana!*"

CHAPTER 4

We Need Frequent and Fabulous Sex

*M*aya was married to Stuart, who was 15 years her junior. Stuart was a photographer for super models. He was accustomed to seeing young, thin, knock-out type ladies on a daily basis. Maya suffered with life-long depression. She was maintained on antidepressants that made her gain weight and caused Stuart to lose interest. The less they made love, the more her depression became non-responsive to drug treatment. They were very close and communicative and discussed all this kindly with each other and thoroughly with me.

Stuart admitted her being so overweight made it difficult for him to desire her. The more she saw he wasn't turned on, the more anxious she became about losing him. The more out of control her eating and the less clean and well dressed she was around the house. They were stuck.

We ultimately balanced both their hormones; hers for brain boosting and appetite control and him for intimacy and desire. She was able to lose weight while on the antidepressants and eventually wean off of them. He was able to have such depth of connection through hormones and exact steps of awakened sex that he longed to connect with her no matter what. His deepening acceptance of her made her relax and she was able to be more in control.

They wrote me a note that they are now happier than they had ever been. Music to my ears!

Sex isn't just fun; it's essential. An essential nutrient is one that your body requires but can't make by itself. Humans are set up to *require* enjoyable sex, the new Vitamin S.

For centuries before humans realized that babies came from sexual intercourse, everyone still had sex. We are set up to make love, our bodies are built to merge. Anatomically, men and women fit together perfectly, and there are many positive health consequences from that merger. And, it turns out, the more *satisfying* the sex, the more *regular* the sex, the more this ups the benefits.

After intensely studying the sex literature and hormone/brain/sex interactions, a pattern emerges. Nature designed sex to care-take the brains of the parents to protect the next generation. Sex is intentionally pleasure-packed so the hormones that are released act as *emotional* glue holding the couple and family together. It is all one big natural sexy scheme to keep life going safely and soundly.

Scientific research on sex

In the past, some societies regarded sex as dangerous to health, but, as with the notions that the world was flat or that tomatoes were poisonous, this old thinking about sex is now known to be completely wrong.

Still, there is a lot of controversy in scientific research surrounding sex, partly because in the past it's been difficult to perform double-blind, placebo-controlled studies on sex. Also, it's the subject itself—it's not easy to get grant money to study sex. But there is a trend happening in the scientific literature that the physical act of sex serves and protects health in both women and men on all levels: body, mind, and spirit. Research has come out exploring and linking sexual well-being with enhanced overall life satisfaction as well as longevity and decreased incidence of illnesses, such as heart disease, cognitive decline and cancer.

Sex, its benefits and importance, is coming out of the bedroom and into the lab.

Four specialists—an endocrinologist, a psychologist, a gynecologist, and a urologist (I know, this sounds like the beginning of a joke, but it isn't)—gave their opinions in the *Journal of Sexual Medicine* in 2009 demonstrating the scientific trend of thought surrounding sex today:

- Sexual activity boosts health benefits in both men and women.

- Sex stimulates healthy testosterone production in both men and women, and this promotes general well-being in both.

- Preliminary research suggests that more frequent sex reduces the risk of prostate and breast cancer.

- Experts suggest that the benefits of satisfying and frequent sexual activity will be so appreciated that sex will be prescribed medically in order to improve general, cognitive, heart, and relationship health of individuals and couples.

We all moan and groan about eating better and exercising more in order to be healthy. Wouldn't it be great if you could accomplish this with sex?

Studies on sex and well-being

Dr. Sonia Davison of the Women's Health Program at Monash University in Australia studied the link between sexual satisfaction and overall well-being. A total of 349 women aged 18 to 65 years were asked how satisfied they were with their sexual life, and then their overall health was monitored. Dr. Davison said, "We found that women who were sexually *dissatisfied* had *lower* overall well-being and lower vitality." In other words, if women weren't getting satisfying sex, and the emphasis is on *satisfying*, they were more fatigued and had less zest for life in general.

Another study looked at women who were sexually active but were having sexual difficulties. The more sexual difficulties they had, the less their overall life satisfaction. The fewer sexual difficulties they had, the better their overall life satisfaction in many arenas. The title of the article says it all: *The Conditional Importance of Sex: Exploring the Association Between Sexual Well-Being and Life Satisfaction*, by Drs. Stephenson and Meston.

These results confirm many previous findings that there is a strong association between sexual well-being and overall life satisfaction.

The better your sex life, the better your outlook! Backed by science.

. . .

If women could look back over their lives
and say that they had satisfying and regular sex
lives, they had healthier blood vessels
and happier overall lives.

. . .

This was also strongly confirmed by a well-known, massive, multi-centered study from the Women's Health Initiative entitled *Sexual Satisfaction and Cardiovascular Disease: The Women's Health Initiative.* They found that if women could look back over their lives and say that they had *satisfying* and *regular* sex lives, they had healthier blood vessels and happier overall lives.

In this study, researchers from Boston University School of Medicine and Boston Medical Center, with collaborators nationwide from numerous prestigious institutions, looked at 93,676 postmenopausal women between the ages of 50 and 79 from 40 clinics for up to 12 years. That's a lot of women from a lot of places. They found that sexually satisfied women have better overall wellness and statistically less plaque (hardening) in their arteries (though during this time frame they did not have lower incidents of actual cardiac events like heart attacks).

Dissatisfaction with sexual activity was modestly associated with plaque build-up in blood vessels, even after controlling for all possible interactions from other life habits, including smoking. Doctors are all looking for ways to keep our blood vessels *dilated* so we'll die later. Sex is one non-pharmaceutical route that has an orgasm (hopefully) at the end of it. In other words, regular *satisfying sex acts like a statin*—a safe and natural (not to mention, fun) one. They also found that older women had more sexual satisfaction than younger women.

This study was begun because sexual dysfunction ("can't get it up") in men is often predictive of heart disease. These investigators in the Women's Health Initiative wanted to see if sexually dissatisfied women with less sex drive had more heart issues, too. As it turns out, they did.

Orgasm reciprocity

When a woman "comes," it is called having an orgasm. When a man comes, it is called ejaculation. I refer to both as orgasm.

Studies are starting to investigate how men and women look at orgasms and their beliefs surrounding them. One study used surveys to collect data from 119 sexually-experienced young British adults; the article was called "*It Feels So Good It Almost Hurts: Young Adults' Experiences of Orgasm and Sexual Pleasure.*" One of the things that came out of the study was the way young Brits were prioritizing *orgasm reciprocity*. This is the contemporary concept that when men and women make love, they both should come.

. . .

Research demonstrates that both men and women truly want each other to come.

. . .

Research demonstrates that both men and women truly want each other to come; it's a dual-job proposition, but with a different timing sequence. Researchers, through surveys and interviews, have demonstrated that both men and women feel *it is the man's responsibility to bring the woman to orgasm first* and *the woman's responsibility is to be open and ready to achieve one* and then to help him.

Salisbury and Fischer explored differences in young adult heterosexual male and female experiences around orgasm, in particular when a woman has difficulty achieving orgasm. This study was based on five male and five female focus groups with three to five participants per group. Transcripts of the discussions were analyzed for emerging themes.

Results showed that when a woman has trouble coming when making love with a man, the most common concern for both men and women is the negative impact this might have on the male partner's ego.

Both male and female participants agreed that men have the *physical responsibility* to stimulate their female partner to orgasm, whether with his penis or his hand or his mouth, while women have the *psychological responsibility* of being mentally prepared to experience the orgasm and to be gentle with the man's ego. That's pretty fascinating.

These researchers also found that the *better and closer the relationship with the partner was perceived to be*, the more pleasurable sex was for both of them, and the more intense the orgasm.

.   .   .

The more you are into your partner, the bigger the bang for your orgasm buck and the more robust the health benefits, especially for the brain.

.   .   .

Quite a number of studies echo this—the more you are into your partner, the bigger the bang for your orgasm buck and the more robust the health benefits, especially for the brain. This is yet another quality reason not to keep hanging on to someone who is not really into you. If he or she is not into you, you are both losing out on your orgasmic karma credits.

It makes sense that part of good life skills is not just having good manners, dressing attractively, or working out, it's also learning how to help your mate reach a satisfying climax. We need to know these things. They don't just download into our brains the day after we are married!

But where do we learn about how to come, how to help someone else come, and how to come in the most enjoyable and beneficial ways possible? Where do we learn how to open up to each other? How to love the other so they won't want or need to look elsewhere?

. . .

Too many of us are still in the sexual dark.

. . .

Most of us were not taught about sex, not told it would be great, not told how to go about it. Many of us were made to feel badly about it. Too many of us are still in the sexual dark. Even if younger people today are more "open" to sexual encounters, it does not mean they are automatically having over-the-moon orgasms! In fact, my medical colleagues and I are often hearing the opposite from younger patients.

Porn can numb real life lovers. Massive sexual freedom may be backfiring and harming the ability to connect. Online dating is like a limitless candy store that promotes an unrealistic pursuit of perfection that keeps us always looking but never committed. There is a need to get back to intimacy basics so unions can be durable, healthy, and ecstatic.

More "Into Each Other" creates more profound orgasms

Science has shown that love is not an absolute necessity to achieve pleasure. But with neuroimaging, being able to look right into the brain at the time of orgasm, studies show beyond a doubt that *a greater emotional connection creates a deeper experience of orgasm,* especially for women.

This suggests that the more you are "into" your mate, and the more you respect them or have a stronger, safer bond of connection, monogamy, or (healthy) marriage, the greater health benefits you get. Orgasms from this type of protected emotional terrain send healthy and protective signals to your brain and all the tissues in your cardiovascular (heart) system.

Using neuroimaging, researchers assessed brain activity of 29 healthy female volunteers. The more women were in love or emotionally close to their partner, the greater the orgasm and the more the satisfaction. But of great brain interest, is that *more areas of the brain* lit up with these *deeper orgasms*. The deeper the orgasms, meaning more *emotionality* combined with *sensuality*, the more healthy brain circulation and activity occurred.

. . .

The deeper the orgasms, meaning more emotionality combined with sensuality, the more healthy brain circulation and activity occurred.

. . .

A study run at four centers looked inside the brain of almost 30 women while orgasming, and graded the emotional depth of their relationship by their rating of how they felt when they saw pictures of their mates.

"In Love" versus "Friends With Benefits"

Being in love and orgasming lights up more and different parts of the brain than having an orgasm without being in love.

In women, being in love lit up an entire brain network involving multiple areas as well as the *angular gyrus*. This is an area of the brain that influences speech. If she loves you, she usually wants to start talking right after having an orgasm. The orgasm lights up that area and now she wants to cuddle, chat, and communicate. He doesn't. His orgasm didn't turn on that area of his brain. No way.

Female orgasms achieved without being in love activate a different area of the brain, called the *left-lateralized insula focus*. It lights up when she moans "OMG." But the more she is into him, the more this specific area *plus* others light up. With each deeper level of emotional connection, when the woman orgasms, more areas light up more intensely. So much so, it's been referred to as a direct indicator of how much pleasure the woman is getting. But that pleasure is influenced by the magical inner workings of her heart.

When a woman is in love, both brain areas light up. The resulting orgasm intensity literally crescendos.

Translated into sex

Guys, how do you turn the pleasure barometer on in your woman's brain? By touch. The authors of this study interpreted the brain scans as demonstrating that when a woman's skin and body are cuddled and touched, her brain area linked with deep satisfaction, the left-lateralized insula focus, is greatly turned on.

So this brain button of pleasure is turned on by either somatic (on the body) touch, or by deeper emotion. So dude! Touch her. Or love her. Or both.

. . .

But those that have flirt within their daily interactions, flourish.

. . .

But when you do touch, have awareness. Be subtle, gentle, and sensual. Do not touch in an absent-minded manner, or too rapidly, or too hard, or like you are hitting the keys on your laptop with speed and lack of exploration. These are less effective ways of touching. The point of your touching is to turn on her brain so you are more into each other.

- Touching a woman's body turns on her testosterone.

- Touching a woman's body turns on brain areas linked with her level of orgasm satisfaction.

- The more you touch her, the greater her pleasure and the more she will want to keep making love with you.

A woman's molecules are complicated. Her biology often requires a slow simmer. Whisper in her ear at breakfast to get her to a full boil at night. Wooing is a life-style. Not 100% of the time of course. But those that have *flirt* within their daily interactions, flourish. This makes molecular sense. Acting on the understanding of how she is hard-wired, and her in return understanding your needs, guarantees unfathomable connection. The authors say these findings show that *being in love* and sexual relationships *without deep love connections,* affect *different* brain regions. The more we are into each other emotionally, the more parts of the brain light up during orgasm, and the bigger the positive brain health jolt.

Translated into more sexy thoughts

Men need to touch *a lot of skin* surface on a woman's body to intensify her experience of pleasure and her brain experience. (This would also hold true for female-female partners, of course.) Men are more commonly focused on direct genital stimulation.

So, women like and need to be touched all over their bodies, and men are more focused on their genitalia. Of course, there are individual differences, and some men may like global touch. Many men (not all) may find touching lots of skin more annoying than a turn-on, especially as the sexual encounter proceeds. Women are turned on by touch. If you aren't really into the lady, gentlemen, at least touch her lovingly and respectfully all over.

The activation of the specific "love" area of the brain, the angular gyrus, demonstrates that *love is different from sex.* Sex has a huge somatic (and emotional) input, but *love is not somatic* (body rather than mind-oriented) *at all.* Rather, love demands a higher cognitive level of involvement. It's in the spirit and the brain.

Orgasms are physical *and* psychological

Another set of researchers wanted to see if pleasure from orgasms was more in the head than in the clitoris or penis. Dr. K. Mah and Dr. Y.

M. Binik investigated male and female participants coming to orgasm either by solitary masturbation or with a partner. There were 350 to 450 individuals in each group. The participants rated their pleasure from solo or partnered experiences. Brain responses were studied by MRI.

This research showed deep orgasmic pleasure and satisfaction were more related to cognitive input than to physical sensory input! Read that sentence over several times. This means that satisfaction takes place more in the brain than below the neck. True pleasure (in the brain) was linked to the overall intensity of orgasm, but not to the specific places on the body—the penis or clitoris—where orgasmsoriginate.

Sex takes place more in the brain than in the body. This is a big part of nature's intention. The more sex, the more our brains get healthy workouts. The smarter we are to take better care of the next generation, and of each other. Nature is strategic.

Sexually Active Life Expectancy (SALE)

Scientists have coined the term SALE, which stands for the average remaining years of sexually active life expectancy. (How many more years are you gonna want to keep doing it?)

For men, SALE used to be about ten years lower than total life expectancy. So if a gent lived to 90 years old, he used to keep wanting sex and buying Viagra and doing it (if he could) until he was 80 years old. But now younger men, even in their 20's, are asking for scripts. If a woman died at 90, she used to stop enjoying and wanting sex when she was 70. Now I also hear this from too many younger women.

In my practice, women commonly tell me that they only *endure* sexual relations for their mates and wish they didn't have to do it at all. They close their eyes and grin and bear it. It seems to me that, over the years, the age range of females dissatisfied with sex is getting younger. This makes me sad. Especially since I see that the women who are still sexually active, either with mates or through solo masturbation, and who aren't isolated or depressed, are the ones with overall happier, healthier lives and brighter brains.

The National Survey of Midlife Development, completed in 1996, looked at 3,000 adults aged 25 to 74, and the National Social Life Health and Aging Project, completed in 2006, involved another 3,000 adults aged 57 to 85. Both studies showed that men stay sexually active longer than women. It seems pretty clear that much of sex is strongly driven by focused and steady testosterone. So for a doctor to leave testosterone replacement out of a women's hormone therapy script, unless it is contraindicated, is missing the "urge" boat.

This difference is most striking as men and women age. In the 75 to 85-year-old group, 40 percent of men remained sexually active compared to 17 percent of women. Data show that men care more about sex than most women. This is one reason men tend to marry younger women, as this creates a more favorable situation for having more sex for a longer period of time. Unless the more mature woman is on hormone replacement, exercises regularly and eats healthfully, which all play a role in keeping hormones humming.

Interest in, quality of, and participation in sex as women age often goes way down compared to men. But multiple studies now affirm a positive association between frequent satisfying sex and later-life health, heart health, brain health and well-being. So too many women are missing out.

However, sexual glitches are not happening just in women. The medical team that I collaborated with on the erectile dysfunction (ED) book is seeing ED in growing numbers of male patients in their twenties and thirties, not just in older males. A urologist, the lead speaker I heard at a hormone conference for MDs and pharmacists, said this is a definite new trend—low blood levels of testosterone and problems with desire and ability in younger men.

Ugh, Irony

Just when we are learning that sex is up there with veggies and exercise, we see a trend of younger men and women not enjoying it. Let alone not being able to do it. To me, this is the height of irony.

Why women (and some men) may not be interested in sex

I speak to patients who come to me for in-depth hormone assessments about their personal relationships and their experience with sex. It is shocking how many women say sex is a big zero for them.

There are lots of reasons they are missing out on sex. Many women just aren't into "it" due to insufficient testosterone blood levels or unbalanced hormones, or their mates no longer have enough libido to engage in sex, or they don't like how their bodies have changed, or they have gained weight and don't want to be touched, or they didn't have a good enough time in their past sexual experiences to keep putting energy into it. Many women today have poor body images due to the media's love affair with perfect bodies, and when women don't like themselves, it's difficult to feel sexy.

Here are more reasons why both men and women might not want sex:

- They are not fully aware of the actual health benefits of sex.

- They still feel squeamish over the idea of sex and guilty for reaping satisfaction from it.

- They have not had effective tools or motivation for achieving mutually satisfying sex.

- Most of them don't know anatomy, such as the G-spot. (I am not aware of sex education classes that teach tools of effective sexual communication or how to find these "pleasure buttons.")

- They may have physical disorders that make sex difficult and unsatisfying, but today there are many technologies to overcome these issues.

- Many are hormonally imbalanced or deficient due to aging, as well as from environmental hormone disruptors, stress, and poor diet.

- Due to medications like antibiotics and daily pain meds (regular use of opioids and even NSAIDs block hormone health), poor dietary choices, or excess alcohol consumption.

- They can also have disrupted gut microbiomes and insufficient digestion, which reduces nutrients and associated hormonal functioning.

- Many are overweight or out of shape and have lost a healthy connection with their own bodies, which translates into less connection with someone else. (*It's hard to have connection with someone else when you don't have it with yourself.*)

- The increase in diabetes and obesity has adversely altered hormones and sex drive.

- Pornography is numbing many to their regular partners and setting up fantastical expectations that ordinary partners can't meet.

- Women are reluctant to speak up about their needs or issues, while men don't create a space where women feel safe to speak up. Women don't have the tools with which to initiate these conversations in a compelling and effective manner.

- Men don't know how to talk, touch, or cuddle. By initiating penile penetration too early, sex can actually hurt. Then she really doesn't want to do it. Who would if it hurts and it isn't turning on their brain?

- Hysterectomies. Some women, after a hysterectomy, will experience diminished pleasure from love-making. During sex, the uterus fills with blood and contracts as orgasm occurs. So the uterus is part of the pleasure a woman's body receives from sex. After hysterectomy, the uterine pleasure input stops. Some women report less pleasure after a hysterectomy, yet some report better sex lives afterwards. Research on intimacy pleasure after hysterectomy is varied. Responses from woman to woman are varied. But any woman can be educated as to how to get her pleasure "back" if she "lost" it after surgery. This book is one of those educational resources.

Sex—the super glue of love

Once men and women start to experience *amazing mutual sex*, their lives are greatly enhanced on all levels, and their relationships mutually improve. Great sex is a "healthy and effective love glue" for long-term relationships because it lights up the part of the brain that has to do with *connection*.

. . .

Great sex is a "healthy and effective love glue" for long-term relationships because it lights up the part of the brain that has to do with connection.

. . .

Four relationship musketeers: Great sex, conversational ability, kindness, and commitment. If you have great ongoing sex with your mate, there is less chance of breaking up than a couple that does not have or enjoy this great intimacy.

In my practice I have seen women who swear up and down that they have never had an interest in sex. Through hormonal testing and balancing, consideration of the nutrients and digestion the hormones lean on, education about the benefits of sex, and the details of how to be "awakened" lovers, their enjoyment explodes. Their orgasms hit high on the Richter scale. Then overall health increases and their eyes sparkle with delight for each other. Relationships reboot!

I have seen women, even in their seventies, eighties, and nineties, not to mention their twenties, suddenly start to have enjoyable and regular sexual activity when they hadn't been doing so for years, if not decades! I know numerous women in their eighties having pleasurable, comfortable *daily* sex with their husbands or with their vibrators. This overflows to all aspects of their lives and relationships on multiple levels.

A walk on the wild side

A patient of mine switched pharmacies, and the new pharmacy's testosterone cream turned out to be much more absorbable than the previous one. Unknowingly, her blood levels of testosterone soared higher than those of most men. Suddenly, she became obsessed with sexual thoughts, with the desire to make love with men just to have release and, strikingly, not to emotionally bond. She was shocked; the experience was so physical and unsentimental. We measured her blood levels and discovered that her testosterone was close to 2000. Most women feel good with blood levels of testosterone around 45 to 80 ng/dL (depending on the lab). Most men feel good with levels between 600 and 900+ ng/dL.

As soon as she stopped taking her testosterone replacement to allow her levels to drift back down to normal (later she would go back on testosterone replacement but at a better dosage for her), all these intense physical sensations ended. She reported all of this to us, in detail, at the clinic. When her testosterone levels spiked high, all her focus was on physical merging and sex, without her heart being involved. Once her testosterone levels came down to normal, sex became as much an emotional as a physical experience once again.

The striking *physicality* of the male hormone testosterone is very real. The striking *emotionality* of the female hormone estrogen is also very real.

How amazing would it be if each man and woman, for one month, got to experience high hormone levels of the opposite sex, to walk in the opposite sex's shoes, so to speak?

Both genders could see and feel how much the male and female hormones rule our experiences of relationships, connection, intimacy and family. And fun. I think this would reduce psychotherapy bills, decrease divorce rates, and boost sexual enjoyment and over all well being for both partners, which is, of course, the true mutual goal!

Health benefits of sex

Sex has multiple benefits for your health. It relieves stress and keeps bodily functions working better, including heart rate, blood pressure, the entire reproductive system, brain chemistry, and signaling and function of the hippocampus. Sex also promotes healthy energy, stamina, and mood. And it has clearly been shown by many studies from different countries that couples that have better sex lives report they have happier relationships.

Sex boosts immunity and gut health

You have a critical player in your immune army called sIgA (secretory immunoglobulin A). It is an antibody (a protein) that lives in moist mucus membranes, such as the mouth, intestinal tract, lungs, and inside the vagina and penis. It boosts immune recognition of foreign invaders, such as bacteria and viruses. Secretory IgA is one of the most active immune players, especially in the lungs and intestinal linings, where much of the immune system flourishes.

The Department of Psychology at Wilkes University had 112 college students report their frequency of sexual encounters, their overall sexual satisfaction, and their relationship status. Then the students had their saliva tested for levels of sIgA. The level of this immune protein in the saliva is reflective of levels in the intestinal tract and lungs and the rest of the body.

The students were divided into four categories based on their sexual frequency: none, infrequent (less than once a week), frequent (one to two times per week), and very frequent (three or more times per week). The results? *More frequent sex boosted better immune function.* Those having sex three or more times a week had 30 percent higher immunoglobulin A levels compared to those with less frequent sex or no sex at all.

In this study it was also interesting to note that the level of immune antibody was not linked to sexual satisfaction or relationship status; it was linked only to the *frequency* of orgasm.

This protective protein is lung and gut protective. So sIgA is also an important part of fighting off lung infections, such as bronchitis and pneumonia. In scientific studies, increased numbers of orgasms in men have been linked to fewer respiratory infections. This protein also is part of maintaining healthy intestinal function as well as helps prevent gut issues like infections and inflammation.

Sex burns calories

You can burn 85 to 200 calories in 30 minutes of sexual activity, depending on how vigorous you are and the duration of exertion. The calories add up. Forty-two half-hour sessions can burn up to 3,570 calories, which is more than enough to lose a pound. Making love for an hour instead of a half hour would be enough calories burned for you to lose one pound within 21 love-making sessions, a bit less than six times a week for a month. Sounds like a great weight maintenance program to me.

Sex reduces the risk of stroke

Some aging men worry that vigorous sex could cause a stroke, like in the movies when a male lover orgasms and suddenly dies on top of his mate (like Goldie Hawn's husband in *Private Benjamin*). But research says otherwise. In a study published in the *Journal of Epidemiology and Community Health*, which followed 914 men for twenty years, scientists found that the frequency of sex was *not* associated with increased stroke. In fact, *more frequent* sex seemed to offer protection *against* stroke. The authors say middle-aged men should not worry about stroking out after an orgasm; regular sex gently helps reduce stroke risk.

The Women's Health Initiative Observational Study and other studies have shown that the more *satisfying* sex a woman has, the more her arteries and heart are protected.

Sex protects against fatal heart attacks

Researchers have found that having sex twice or more a week *reduces* the risk of fatal heart attack by half, compared with men who had sex less than once a month.

Sex also promotes optimal *heart rate variability* (HRV). HRV is a marker of the how "in sync" your heart and nervous system are. The healthier your HRV, the better your overall health. HRV reflects heart rate fluctuations in response to a variety of subtle demands on your body, like breathing. Resting HRV is run mainly by the calming parasympathetic nervous system. Optimal HRV levels are associated with better sexual functioning, better emotional responses, happier moods in both men and women, and living longer and healthier. Regular and satisfying sex lives are linked to healthier HRVs in both males and females.

Sex is cardiovascular exercise. So sex exercises the blood vessels and hearts in both women and men. Sex improves strength, flexibility, muscle tone, and cardiovascular conditioning. It's like an intimacy cross-fit.

Sex relieves stress

Stress can make blood vessels constrict and then blood pressure rises. This is called blood pressure reactivity. It happens with *the white coat syndrome*. A doctor walks into the room and you see this as a stress and your blood pressure spikes. Folks with high blood pressure reactivity are said to be at higher risk for *hypertension* (sustained high blood pressure) down the road. Well, sex, penile-vaginal sex that is, reduces blood pressure reactivity. In a German study, people exposed to stress but who had practiced penile-vaginal sex for two weeks prior, had less blood pressure spiking.

In other words, it's easier for your blood vessels to "chill out" if you keep getting some intimacy!

Sex and hormones

Testosterone in both males and females and estrogen levels in women get a boost from regular sexual activity. In men, testosterone protects the heart, bones, and muscles and, in women, estrogen protects the heart, brain, bones, memory, and skin tone. Cuddling makes women's bodies make more testosterone and want to keep cuddling. Then the rise of estrogen during sex makes a women more responsive to touch as well as upping her desire to connect more with her man.

. . .

Testosterone in both males and females and estrogen levels in women get a boost from regular sexual activity.

. . .

Men can start to over-produce estrogen (in ratio to their testosterone) as they age and accumulate more fat cells (fat cells make estrogen). Their estrogen levels increase while their testosterone levels drop. They develop breasts. Their risk of prostate cancer rises. They loose that manly essence. To the rescue is *regular* sex which helps keep a healthier ratio between these two hormones. But as we age, intimacy might not be enough and hormone balancing and replacement by prescription may become a necessary part of the solution.

Sex and prostate cancer

Regular sex reduces symptoms of benign prostatic hypertrophy disease. This is enlargement of the prostate gland that is usually due to inadequate circulation from too little exercise or love-making, not due to a serious issue like cancer. Frequent sex helps prevent the issue in the first place.

Regular sex house-cleans the prostate. A 2003 Australian study found that out of 2,338 men, those who ejaculated five times or more a week were a third *less* likely to develop prostate cancer by age 70 than those who ejaculated fewer times a week. The lead author of the study, Dr. Graham G. Giles, concluded that regular ejaculation appears to flush cancer-causing and damaging toxins out of the prostate, thereby protecting prostatic tissue.

The men in this study who ejaculated 21 times per month (this is equal to having sex/orgasm five to six times each week) showed a statistical reduction in prostate cancer over a lifetime.

An increase of three ejaculations per week throughout one's lifetime is associated with a 15 percent *decrease* in the risk of prostate cancer.

Men who recalled having four or more ejaculations per week in their younger years (twenties, thirties, and forties) had one-third less risk of developing prostate cancer compared to men who reported fewer ejaculations per week in their earlier and middle years.

The largest study on the protective effects of frequent orgasms in men came out of Yale. Jennifer R. Rider ScD, MPH, presented her results at a urology conference in 2014. This prospective study followed 32,000 men across 18 years of life and documented who got prostate cancer. This was compared to how the men lived—the foods they consumed or if they smoked or not, and how often they orgasmed.

The scientists found that *frequency of orgasm* throughout a man's life course was *inversely* associated with his risk of prostate cancer. The more men ejaculated, the healthier their prostate and the less often they got prostate cancer.

Another frequency study came out of Canada (University of Montreal and INRS, Institut Armand-Frappier). Men who never had sexual intercourse were twice as likely to have prostate cancer compared to men who had. Men who had over 20 women lovers in their lifetime had 28% reduction of all types of prostate cancer and 19% reduction in the most aggressive type!

More frequent sex rinses toxins out of the prostate. This promotes better prostate health.

What about homosexuals? Scientists from the University of Montreal's School of Public Health tracked 3,208 men (part of the Montreal Prostate Cancer & Environment Study). The data showed that if a gay man had sex in his lifetime with one other male, it didn't increase his risk of getting prostate cancer. But if a man had sex with more than 20 different men, he was twice as likely to be diagnosed with prostate cancer. This is only a single study, but it's pretty fascinating. Why would that be? At this point we do not know.

The authors summarized their findings:

- Having had more than 20 female sexual partners was associated with decreased prostate cancer risk.

- Having had more than 20 male sexual partners was suggestive of greater prostate cancer risk.

- No links were found between sexually transmitted infections and the risk of prostate cancer.

Sex and breast cancer

. . .

Here it is again, maleness protecting femaleness.

. . .

Women who regularly made love and were exposed to semen on a frequent basis (unprotected love-making) for at least 20 years had one-tenth the breast cancer risk compared to women who never had intercourse! The authors, from the Institut National de la Santé et de la Recherche Médicale, Institut Gustave Roussy, Villejuif, France, said that direct contact with semen was the main protective factor. Here it is again, *maleness* protecting *femaleness*.

Sex keeps you looking younger

An active sex life promotes looking younger than your chronological age. Look what folks go through with facelifts and chemical peels, when here we are talking of the big O as an intimacy cosmetic procedure!

Intercourse increases levels of both male hormones in both males and females. We have already learned that it increases the male hormone testosterone. It also increases the other male hormone, DHEA (dehydroepiandrostone). This hormone, in both men and women, has been linked to shiny, glowing complexions (it boosts sebaceous cell secretions that give skin healthy moisture). DHEA promotes younger-looking skin, shiny, healthy eyes, and a perky libido.

Semen contains two estrogens that are linked to promoting healthier collagen levels in the skin, especially the face.

Dr. David Weed, a clinical neuropsychologist, headed an 18-year-long study on 3,500 people called the *Super-Young Project*. This study examined people who look and feel ten years younger than their chronological age, and the researchers tried to identify which factors were responsible. Why did these older people look so much younger than many of their cronies?

Through extensive questionnaires and interviews, it was discovered that a powerful promoter of looking and feeling younger was *frequency* of sex.

In one of the experiments, judges looked at participants through a one-way mirror and guessed their ages. The subjects who were consistently rated seven to twelve years younger than their real age were labeled "super-young." On the average, the super-young looking participants reported having sexual intercourse three times a week in comparison to the age-appropriate-appearing group who reported sex an average of twice a week.

Vanity is one of my favorite sins. If for no other reason than more frequent sex makes us look younger and more attractive, this is yet another reason to visit the boudoir more often.

Sex fights insomnia

Make love at night. Ha! Or for that afternoon nap!

Sex improves sperm quality

This does not just mean the number of sperm, but their ability to swim, mingle, and mate with eggs.

Sex may decrease depression

If no condom is used, the testosterone in semen may decrease depression and even suicide attempts, and boost emotional quality of life in women. Studies on college age women show that women regularly engaging in penile-vaginal sex used less depressants and made less suicide attempts compared to women making love regularly with protection. Semen, remember, contains positive brain mood boosters.

Sex is fun

Life is not just about hard work, and fun is not flippant. *Healthy sexual fun is as necessary as food and water.* Sex is a healthy, natural way to recharge the body's batteries on all levels—*body, mind, and spirit.*

If you are in a relationship and one of you stops making love and the other of you wishes this were not the case, both of you *must* discuss, deal with, and heal this situation. You cannot have a healthy, lasting relationship and pretend this elephant is not living in and disrupting your bedroom and entire home. Even if one person needs, for whatever reason, to not engage in intimacy for a period of time, this needs to be mutually discussed, explained and agreed upon, to keep the relationship healthy. And to keep the door open down the road for recreating mutually satisfying connection when the time is right.

CHAPTER 5

The Condom Conundrum

*M*arian had a fetish about getting a sexually transmitted disease even though she and her boyfriend had been living together for seven years. Kevin swore he was faithful, but just to be safe, Marian insisted on using condoms. Marian suffered with severe anxiety and insomnia. She was addicted to Valium. She had been on it for years and it no longer really helped with these issues, but when she attempted to stop taking it, her problems got worse.

I explained to Marian that sex with a condom had her losing out on the anti-depressive and calming molecules it could offer. Marian was shocked. Kevin was amazed. I emphasized that the psychological and health benefits only occur when sex is regular. So they both made a commitment to date and mate at least twice a week if not more.

Within two months Marian's anxiety was gone. She slept so soundly she snored, but Kevin couldn't complain. Better yet, she was finally able to slowly wean off Valium. They got engaged and set a date.

I'm fascinated by the chemical complexity of semen. Until recently, scientists alleged that the major purpose of semen was to feed and protect sperm on their way toward searching out and mingling with an egg (fertilization). But now, scientific evidence seems to show that semen "gifts" women the experience of more stable happiness in return for women opening themselves up to the potential act of creation or just plain being open to another of nature's creations, the "other" human being.

Ejaculation and semen

What's that stuff coming out of the penis when a man makes love? Ejaculation is the normal release of liquid from the penis during the sexual response. During sex, semen builds up in thin tubes called ejaculatory ducts. When sexual arousal is so powerful that there is no turning back (called *ejaculatory inevitability*) rhythmic contractions in a group of muscles, in the prostate and pelvis (peritoneal muscles) and the shaft of the penis, become uncontrollable. At first these contractions are at 0.8-second intervals, propelling and spurting semen during ejaculation. After three or four contractions, intervals between spurts lengthen and the intensity calms down.

Semen is the white stuff that spurts out of the penis during ejaculation. It *may* contain sperm. This semen, emitted from the urethra during ejaculation, is milky and shiny. Sperm has the appearance of gemstone opals, so the more sperm the semen contains, the more opalescent it appears. Sperm can make up from 1 to 10 percent of semen, and this composition varies from guy to guy.

Semen doesn't start with the initial part of ejaculation; it starts a few seconds after ejaculatory inevitability. However, don't think that pulling out immediately is a good way to prevent getting pregnant; it isn't. *You can't time the release of semen.*

When seminal fluid is ejaculated into a woman, she gets a *physiologic shot glass full* of mood-elevating, anti-depressive, immune-boosting and hormone-zesting substances. Women who regularly make love with men (without condoms) have been shown to have less depression and anxiety and a better quality of life. Why is that? Look what's inside semen.

Semen is better than an over the counter one-a-day

All that white stuff during ejaculation is actually a multi-mineral, protein-rich, hormone-boosting, low-carb (Paleo friendly!) stimulus that a man gifts a woman while making love. It can enhance her mood, brain, and whole body health because seminal fluid is pure gold, move over Centrum one-a-days. Seminal fluid contains approximately 50 compounds! Examples are: free amino acids (building blocks of protein), fructose, enzymes, phosphorylcholine (helps sperm motility), testosterone, two estrogens, prolactin (hormone of satisfaction), prostaglandins, and many minerals, especially zinc.

. . .

Semen contains two female sex estrogens—estrone and estradiol—in the same exact form that the human body has always used (known as bioidentical hormones).

. . .

Semen contains two female sex estrogens—estrone and estradiol—in the same exact form that the human body has always used (known as bioidentical hormones). Semen also contains a variety of mood-elevating compounds, such as endorphins, prolactin, oxytocin, thyrotropin-releasing hormone, and serotonin, the well-known mood elevator in both brains (the head and in the gut).

Certain gut diseases, like irritable bowel syndrome (IBS), are treated by drugs or nutraceuticals that boost serotonin. So instead of taking a pill a day to treat your depression or irritable bowel syndrome, you might try regular afternoon quickies.

A special note on semen and zinc

Semen is a natural multi-mineral, with an emphasis on *zinc*. Zinc is a mineral that enables 300 critical enzymes and over 1,000 factors (called transcription factors) to assist genes in their magical work. Zinc is the most abundant mineral found in the human brain, especially in the

73

hippocampus. When men and women make love regularly, with exchange of fluids, women get more zinc exposure in their brain tissues. This is a good thing! Zinc has been shown to enhance cognitive function of the brain.

Locally, zinc protects sperm by killing any bacteria that might harm it. But zinc also protects the woman by acting as a powerful immune enhancer and antioxidant. And *zinc makes all hormones work more efficiently*. Even if your blood levels of testosterone or estrogen are within normal range, if you are deficient in zinc, your hormones might not work optimally. Your hormones need zinc. If your zinc levels are low, you might suffer low desire or performance, even if you are taking hormone replacement therapy or even if your blood or saliva or urine levels of hormones test optimally.

When hormones swim into a waiting receptor to receive their message, zinc atoms in the shape of a fold so they are literally called "zinc fingers" grab the hormone and connect it to where it needs to go in the genes to deliver the hormone's messages. So getting a bit of zinc on a daily basis helps hormones function optimally for a woman. Once again, this is *maleness protecting femaleness*.

The prostate stores zinc, and half of its reserves are used up during ejaculation. When the ejaculate goes into the vagina, the zinc is absorbed into the woman and aids in the egg and sperm uniting. The zinc in the ejaculate contributes to her zinc stores and her overall hormonal functioning, as well as her moods and her immune functioning. The zinc from sperm is part of what puts a spring in her step the next morning.

With males, they lose a bit of zinc each time they ejaculate. Thus a man has to be consuming and digesting zinc regularly in his diet (through foods like oysters, salmon, shrimp, organic beef, kidney beans, flax seeds, spinach, cashews, pumpkin seeds, dark chocolate, soybeans, sesame seeds, wheat germ, shitake mushrooms, and chickpeas) to replenish the approximately 134 mcg (.134 mg) of zinc lost during each ejaculation. If he is not eating enough zinc rich foods, or digesting them, yet regularly making love, his hippocampus starts to get "low" in zinc and his hormones that feed this tissue can't signal like they should.

So yes, a man can have so much sex his brain functions less well, unless he keeps up his stores of zinc. A man can fornicate his brains out, so to speak. So, it's a good idea to take a multi-mineral that contains zinc to keep your bases and your brain covered.

The vaginal sponge

Vaginal tissue is highly absorptive. Like a sponge. It's richly endowed with blood and lymph vessels waiting to soak up whatever enters inside. Vaginal tissue has been show to easily absorb many of the substances in semen, such as zinc, testosterone, estrogen, follicle stimulating hormone, luteinizing hormone, prolactin, and a number of different prostaglandins.

Testosterone is absorbed more quickly through the vagina than through the skin. Research has shown that numerous biological products contained in seminal fluid, including the hormones and prostaglandins, can be measured in the female's bloodstream within several hours after ejaculation.

This is one reason that many doctors now recommend hormonal replacement therapy delivery through the vagina (transmucosal delivery) as the hormones are rapidly absorbed with *fewer health risks* compared to other *delivery modes,* such as swallowing, slathering on skin, or melted inside the cheek. Nature intended the vagina to be exposed to hormones and be set up to absorb them and deliver them to the bloodstream. (I discuss this at length in *Safe Hormones, Smart Women* and its upcoming revision *Safe Hormones.*)

Repeated ejaculations

The ability to have repeated ejaculations—one after the other—begins to decline right after puberty ends (when the male body now has all its hair, manly voice, and secondary sex changes). Most adult men experience only one ejaculation within a one- to two-hour period. Some can have two ejaculations during this same time frame. It is rare, but some men may be able to have three or four during this same period. Their names should be on milk cartons!

The act of ejaculation is healthy for men. The more ejaculations, the less heart disease and longer life span men may expect. An investigation published in the *British Medical Journal* in 1997 showed that of one thousand men, those who experienced orgasms at least twice a week had a *50 percent reduced mortality* at earlier ages compared to men who had orgasms less than once a month. At a ten-year follow-up, the group of men with two or more orgasms per week had *half the number of fatal coronary events* (such as heart attack and stroke) compared with the men with lower orgasm frequency.

This shows that more *frequent* ejaculations protect the heart and promote longer life!

Having sex often also ensures healthier sperm. The more frequently a man ejaculates, the more his sperm-production machinery has to keep up with the demand. It's a practice-makes-perfect kind of thing. It takes roughly 48 days for new sperm to form and another 14 for it to fully mature, so this process is constantly churning away. Storing sperm by avoiding ejaculation, which in the past was mistakenly thought to build better sperm counts, can actually decrease the sperm motility.

It's the density of sperm in each ejaculate that diminishes with frequent orgasms; the quality of sperm does not get worse, it gets better. With more frequent orgasms, sperm are healthier—improved agility, swimming power, and quality of inner fatty acids. And of note, once sperm enter a woman's body, they can live (stay viable) within the female reproductive tract for up to five days after sex, which explains why the rhythm method is so hit-and-miss. But it may be that healthier sperm stay viable longer and may contribute to enhanced fertility.

Sperm and fertility

Most men mistakenly believe that the more semen they make, the more fertile they are. Not so. A single ejaculation varies in its content of sperm. It can contain anywhere between 40 million to 600 million sperm, depending on the volume of the ejaculate but also on how long it has been since the last ejaculation.

A typical ejaculation can travel some distance—the average is seven to ten inches—but some have a force that allows the semen to travel up to three feet. Nature is about the next generation and created that powerful force to get those sperm into the woman.

Ejaculation is preceded by a release of one or two drops of clear fluid from the Cowper's glands (two small glands beneath the prostate). This fluid is very *alkaline*. Nature puts it here to protect the sperm by neutralizing the acidity from any remaining urine in the urethra. If the man recently urinated, the semen, being alkaline, is a backup system to insure a better environment for potential reproduction (again safeguarding the next generation).

Semen as an antidepressant.

When women come together with men and open themselves up to receiving their sperm (in a relationship safe to do so without a condom) and start the cascade steps of *potential* reproduction, they are "protected" *emotionally* as well as *physically*.

. . .

Sperm is like a mini-dose of bioidentical hormone therapy.

. . .

Sperm is like a mini-dose of bioidentical hormone therapy. Semen contains many hormones and prostaglandins that have been called "feel-good" molecules as they are linked to better mood, happiness, and less depression in a large number of studies. Because the vagina acts like a physiologic sponge and demonstrates a high degree of absorptiveness, and semen contains so many mood-elevating compounds, Drs. Gallup and Burch and Steven Platek wondered if women exposed to semen might experience less depression and have better moods, compared to women exposed to less semen from use of condoms.

Women are known to be three to five times more susceptible to depression compared to men. But, these scientists pondered, "*Do women who are less exposed to semen have more depression than women who are regularly exposed to semen?*" They designed a scientific analysis to evaluate this. Gallup, Burch, and Platek surveyed 293 college women at the State University of New York in Albany, New York, about their intercourse habits and use of condoms and then tested their moods by the Beck Depression Inventory, a standard test of mood.

It turned out that women who had *more* exposure to semen had *less* depression, and this result was *statistically significant*, meaning that it occurred beyond random chance. The investigators also found that women exposed to more semen (through regular sex without condoms) reported fewer suicide attempts compared to women whose lovers used condoms.

The authors wisely wanted to make sure that the decreased depression with regular semen exposure wasn't actually due to these women being in committed relationships and thus feeling more emotionally stable. By asking specific questions in the survey, the authors were able to show that this was not what is called a "confounding variable" contributing to the improved mood; rather, the exposure to semen was the effective link.

The scientists say that their results suggest that females who have sex without condoms, and are therefore more likely to have mood-boosting components from that semen in their reproductive tract that eventually finds it way to their brain, have significantly fewer depressive symptoms than those who use condoms (or have less sex). Also, the more that women avoided condoms, the more often they had sex. The authors wondered if this was because sex boosted the moods of these women. And does this say that we are meant to have more satisfying sex in the confines of a committed relationship?

Ejaculation for better moods

Glutamate and GABA (gamma-aminobutryic acid) are signaling hormones, or neurotransmitters in the central nervous system, including the brain. Balance between them, like in everything else, is essential. Too much glutamate and one can be anxious, depressed, wired/tired, or have trouble recovering from chronic health problems. Too little GABA and one can't calm down or achieve restorative sleep and might have to live on anti-anxiety medications.

· · ·

More connecting sex, less aggression.

· · ·

After sex, men have that lilt in their step; they feel better. This isn't a line of bull—it's chemistry. Regular ejaculations are a gatekeeper in that they help maintain a healthier *balance* between the excitatory glutamate and the calming/inhibitory GABA in males. More connecting sex, less aggression.

Here's another fascinating note: Elevated levels of glutamate have been linked with serious diseases of the eye, such as glaucoma. So regular sex protects eyes, not the other way around as masturbation myths of the past suggested.

In daily human life, many things seem to come down to money, although some still say it all comes down to love. In nature, it all comes down to the survival of the next generation. Semen, sex, and sperm all keep this intrinsically in mind.

Heterosexual intercourse without condoms

There is a massive body of peer review science (the kind that is reviewed and given the okay by highly respected peers) comparing mood, brain, and health benefits depending on what "style" of sex we have. Meaning, how we do it. Steve Brody PhD is a psychological scientist and couple's therapist (out of the University of the West of Scotland, School of Social Sciences, in the UK) who has published an enormous body of original research as well as research reviews of many other scientists. Dr. Brody wrote an exceptionally extensive review of the science comparing love configurations, published in 2010, called, *"The Relative Health Benefits of Different Sexual Activities."*

Dr. Brody writes that when the penis enters the vaginal vault, called *penile–vaginal intercourse,* the rubber meets the road, although it's best when no rubber is used! Dr. Brody showed that when mutual orgasm is achieved without condom barrier protection, the benefits are much more profound than when orgasm is achieved by any other means (clitoral stimulation or by masturbation). The most documented benefits on brain, mood, and against premature death and cancer come with penile-vaginal stimulation without condoms blocking the exchange of fluids.

In a 25-year follow-up study by a gerontologist (one who studies aging), men lived longer the more they enjoyed penile-vaginal sex regularly with their partners. In the Women's Health Initiative Observational Study, if a woman could look back over her sexual memories over her lifetime and say she enjoyed them, and they were penile-vaginal penetration style, these women lived longer (and happier).

In a 10-year study on almost a thousand men from Wales from the University of Bristol, the more orgasms men had, the lower their age of death from all causes, but especially heart disease. Sexual activity, frequency (and especially penile-vaginal intercourse) was concluded to be a major protector of male health. At least twice weekly was needed for this degree of health and heart protection.

I have NO judgment against masturbation, same sex partners, or other styles of sex. *I am a reporter of the science.* Any route of connection and release has benefits and can boost pleasure. And in *no* way do I mean to encourage "unsafe" sex. But the findings from research do suggest that nature *wants* us to be monogamous, not promiscuous. Just be aware that using a condom inhibits the exchange of critical mood- and hormone-boosting natural compounds. Nature set up greater benefits when sex is shared with someone you love and respect, and with whom you can make love safely without condoms most of the time.

The Birth Control Dilemma

As you have learned, intimacy has health and brain benefits. All forms of intimacy serve human health, even cuddling without the act of penetration or love-making with a condom. But the ideal sexual *togetherness* is making love with your committed beloved when you can share all there is to be shared without barriers like condoms.

But that is often not possible.

It would be irresponsible of me not to mention birth control, and what a conundrum it is.

According to the Centers for Disease Control and Prevention, oral contraceptives are the most common type of birth control, used by 11.7 million women. They are convenient. They are effective. They help prevent pregnancy. But they have potential long-term serious health effects that too few docs or women know about. And birth control pills do not protect against many serious health issues like STDs (from herpes to worse) and AIDS.

Too few women know about the shadow side of oral contraceptives. And docs have differing opinions about what is best to do. Very few understand that the synthetic hormones used in birth control pills are endocrine disruptors that are not without some serious problems.

Birth control pills rinse many critical nutrients out of the body. Every drug rinses at least one nutrient out of the body, but more than any other drug, birth control pills rinse out more essential nutrients, such as folate. If a baby is born while the mom is on the pill (it can happen) or soon after she stops taking them, the baby is often deficient in these nutrients. For example, a baby has a higher risk of being born with spina bifida unless the mother supplemented with adequate folate while on the pill to offset the loss of folate caused by the pill.

Few docs tell women this.

Birth control pills disrupt estrogen genes. Estrogen genes need to work well throughout your entire life. Especially, as you have learned, for brain health. Disruption of these genes, even for a short time, has been shown to have far-reaching effects. This can happen in the adult woman or to a baby born to a woman on the pill or just having gotten off of it.

Birth control pills can ruin desire. In a randomized and controlled human trial (this means the information is scientifically powerful), the most popular oral contraceptive used in Sweden that contains a synthetic progestin called levonorgestrel and a synthetic estrogen named ethinyl estradiol, significantly reduced desire, arousal and pleasure in some women. This was published in the Journal of Clinical Endocrinology and Metabolism in August, 2016.

Birth control pills create a false physiologic pregnancy. A growing number of nutritionally-oriented experts agree. Dr. Norman Shealy, a neurosurgeon turned medical nutritionist, says the use of birth control, after taking pills for a year or more, damages the cross-talk between the brain and hormones in the body. (Dr. Shealy taught this information at a 40-hr CEU course I took from him at his college in Missouri in 2014.)

I specialize in treating with nutrition many complex patients who are not getting well through regular medical means. While doing intakes of patient history, I have seen a repetitive association with the long-term use of birth control pills and the onset of disease. I then have to use lots of nutritional, herbal, and glandular, if not hormonal "magic," to reboot the HPA axis (hypothalamic, pituitary, adrenal axis cross-talk).

In human trials from respected institutions, birth control pills have been linked to an increased risk of plaque in the arteries and heart disease, even in young women, as well as to stroke and breast cancer. They have also been linked to worsened seizures in women with epilepsy. They have been linked to less uterine and ovarian cancer, but with more allergies and migraines in some women and less in others.

Birth control pills are one of the main causes of stroke in perimenopausal ladies. I see many gynecologists give these synthetic hormones to women in their late thirties and forties, when this is a definite no-no; only bioidentical forms of hormone replacement must be used to balance hormones at that age.

Birth control pills are recommended for female issues other than protection from pregnancy, such as for PCOS, heavy bleeding during periods, and migraines. But there are many natural answers that are better for these conditions without the long-term issues that women are not informed of (and many docs don't know about).

Birth Control Pills Don't Protect

When you date someone and don't know their health history or if they are truly monogamous with you, birth control pills are not enough. You have to add condoms to the equation to safeguard against diseases that can be spread by unprotected sex, let alone worry about pregnancy.

So, it's a tough decision, as the pill allows women and men to enjoy the closest of intimacies, usually without condoms. Nothing surrounding intimacy, sexual relations, and hormones is simple. When I discussed birth control options with various gynecologists, I got answers that ranged all over the map, including "Tell her to keep an aspirin between her knees!"

So what is a fertile female to do?

Diaphragms tend not to get used often enough and certainly lack sexual spontaneity. Cervical caps are too awkward for many women. IUDs (intrauterine devices) are very convenient. But commonly used ones contain a synthetic progestin, which can be linked to bone loss when a woman gets older and other health issues like stroke. It is the synthetic progestin that has been most linked to an increased risk of breast cancer and other woes.

The copper IUD, which doesn't contain hormones, is good for many women. Not all. I have seen some of my patients with inflammatory conditions (like inflammatory bowel disease), get worse from the copper component in the IUD. But it is the unmedicated IUD at the time of writing this book that seems the most sensible. But once in a while a woman can get pelvic inflammatory disease (PID) from this mechanical barrier method. And you still are not protected against STDs and AIDs.

Even condoms have their problems with how they are used. In reality, condoms are supposed to be used with spermicidal gels to make them more effective and to then also protect against these STDs. But how often is that done?

This book is introducing the idea that sex without condoms provides maximum health and brain benefits. But all forms of intimacy help boost health, immune, and brain function. Even cuddling boosts levels of testosterone in females.

However, fact is fact. Most sexual relationships require some form of birth control or protection from disease. About the only relationships I can think of that unprotected sex would work for *consistently* are a young couple looking to get pregnant or after menopause, when both partners are trusted to be totally monogamous.

When needed, use the best protection you can. Sometimes you need to be on a 24/7 birth control. And sometimes when you know you are safe physically and emotionally, get really intimate without condoms. It's your life, your lifestyle, and your intentions that dictate your needs and answers.

It is not within the scope of this book to address the issue of birth control in detail. I hope you have an *integrative* health team with whom you can discuss all these issues. This team should understand the shadow side of allopathic birth control pills and synthetic hormones. The estrogen used in birth control pills is a synthetic one. It is an endocrine disruptor. The pill may prevent pregnancy and stop your heavy periods, but it may increase the risk of estrogen receptor alpha-driven diseases down the road. You need a team that has a bigger understanding of hormones and their signals and what may be the best answer for you.

Considering that long-term birth control pills may cause more headaches than they fix, up the possibility of allergies, rinse the body of vitamin C, folate, and other nutrients, why isn't finding new non-chemical means of birth control a top research priority? Whatever happened to my old favorite—the sponge? It wasn't just Elaine on Seinfeld that loved that form of birth control; I did, too. Or what about those old things I used to use after the sponge disappeared—the tampon-like insertion of spermicide?

Use common sense, ask lots of questions, and review all your options.

As far as my general recommendation, it is to use the non-hormonal IUD, which is one of the most effective contraceptive methods available at this time. It is also easily reversed. Its failure rate is less than 1%. That is about its risk of pelvic infection and inflammatory disease. But there is no 100% answer. Some integrative docs recommend the vaginal ring, but that's if you can get it with a non-synthetic estrogen, at least in my book. I know this seems like a lot to take in about a very delicate subject, but hormones are the most powerful signaling molecules in your body. If you are going to put something inside you and leave it in, you should do some research. Your grandmother's generation did everything the doc said to do, which got us all into trouble. Don't continue that deer-in-the-headlights behavior as a patient!

Condom effectiveness

The male condom is 98% effective, *if used perfectly*. But the failure rate goes up to 18% with "typical" use, such as putting on the condom partway through intercourse, removing it before intercourse is over, failing to look for damage before use, and failing to leave space at the tip of the condom for semen. An 18% failure rate means that out of 100 women who rely only on condoms for birth control, 18 will get pregnant.

Four out of five women use the pill because they do not know most of what is written in this section. For example, here is an eye opener. Researchers from Ghent University in Belgium looked at 1,301 apparently healthy women between the ages of 25 and 55 who had previously used oral contraceptives, half of whom used them for 13 years or more. Women who had used the pills had an unexpected increase in artery-clogging plaque in key blood vessels supplying the brain and legs. *Women had a 20 to 30 percent increase in plaque for every 10 years they had taken oral contraceptives.* They presented their findings at the American Heart Association scientific sessions in Orlando, Florida, in 2007.

So the debate surrounding birth control pills and birth control is very real. That's why I called this section what I did. A dilemma.

Lesbians

The *McClintock effect* is the name for the phenomenon that occurs when clusters of women get in sync with each other. This refers to groups of reproductive-age women who live or work together (in college dorms, the military, monasteries, all-female workplaces, etc.) and whose menstrual periods start to get synchronized over time (meaning they start their periods around the same time each month). The scientific explanation is that the women detect each other's pheromones, subtle but powerful scent compounds, which influence women's hormonal menstruation time.

But the stickler is that studies have demonstrated that women who have sex only with other women don't exhibit this McClintock effect. Two evolutionary psychologists at the State University of New York, Drs. Gordon Gallup and Rebecca Burch, researched this phenomenon. These scientists found that an identifiable difference between lesbians and heterosexual women regarding the McClintock effect is that hetero ladies are exposed to semen, while lesbians aren't. The vaginas of the women who were making love with men and getting exposed to semen absorbed compounds from the seminal fluid that affected their pheromones.

The happiness quotient

Happiness—satisfaction with your life and relationships in general—has been shown to occur more in couples that regularly practice unprotected sex compared to couples where the partners either use condoms or frequently practice masturbation rather than sex with each other.

In a study of 2,810 Swedes, researchers found two scenarios that are linked to more happiness: penile-vaginal penetration and how often it was shared without condoms. The happiest women (most life satisfied), made love with their man without condoms and experienced vaginal orgasm, compared to women who only had orgasm through clitoral manipulation, either by their man or by solo masturbation. The name of this study is "*Satisfaction (sexual, life, relationship, and mental health) is associated directly with penile-vaginal intercourse, but inversely with other sexual behavior frequencies."*

Drs. Brody and Costa concluded that frequent penile-vaginal sex is linked to being happy sexually, to being healthy, and to having more well-being in all aspects of life. They concluded that masturbation is inversely related to these life benefits. (This doesn't mean that a happy, well-adjusted single person who masturbates will have adverse outcomes. We will discuss this more at length later.)

Condoms

Condoms, those life-saving devices, protect against disease, but they also block sensation, the deeper intimacy that comes from that sensation, and the magical exchange of fluids and energy that are meant to occur naturally. Replicated research shows that condoms create poorer emotional integration in some lovers. That study really astounded me.

In 2010, Portuguese participants had their emotional health evaluated and compared to the ways these couples achieved orgasm, including whether or not they used protection. The study concluded that couples who had regular penile-vaginal sex and orgasms *without condoms* reported less negative emotional issues (labeled as immature and neurotic defenses) compared to couples who regularly used condoms.

Freud (whose work I studied when getting my psychoneurology BA at the U of Michigan) was one of the first to say that condoms impair intimacy and sensation, which can (emphasis on *can*, not *will*) lead to less satisfying orgasms, and even promote neurotic behavior. Of course, Freud was the father of all things neurotic!

Research from early Kinsey Sex Reports linked marital happiness with the woman being stimulated directly by the penis without use of condoms. In a Swedish study, men had better relationship satisfaction and used masturbation less often when they had more frequent unprotected penile-vaginal sex.

Sperm is about the next generation, so whatever can safeguard sperm is significant. It turns out that *penile-vaginal sex is more sperm protective* than other forms of sex.

Two human studies produced these findings. Sperm was studied every which way (number, shape, and mobility) and samples were compared from men who masturbated versus those who achieved orgasm by penile-vaginal sex. Volume of sperm and its fluids, sperm count, sperm motility, and percentage of well-shaped healthy sperm were all greater in the samples from men who orgasmed by vaginal penetration compared to masturbation. One group of researchers said that orgasming by penile-vaginal penetration promoted healthier sperm as well as prostate function.

Who'd a thunk it?

The more we come together, feel, connect, and commit deeply, the better sex takes care of us. This suggests sensible and safe relationships, marriages, and nuclear families are where nature intended to take those of us that want to go there.

CHAPTER 6

Testosterone—Benefits & Controversies

Mark was a man's man. He had been military all his life,
still had perfectly polished shoes and prided himself on
walking, talking, and making love like a manly man.
But when he turned 67 years old, things changed. His motivation tanked. He
thought about doing things, but couldn't do them. He felt overwhelmed, which
made him anxious. His wife had seen me and had her hormones balanced.
She was back in the game and wanted Mark back in the sack. In the past that
would have lit Mark's fire, but now her desire seemed intimidating.

He went to the VA for all his health concerns. Mark's VA doc ran his testosterone level, which was down near the bottom but still within the normal
range. So the doc said Mark's T was good to go. He also told Mark that testosterone wasn't healthy for the heart anyway. So Mark suffered until he came
to see me.

I retested Mark's testosterone, as well as his estrogen levels. Turned out his
estrogen was sky high, so the ratio of his estrogen to his testosterone was off.
In essence, Mark was being feminized. He also drank several beers a day,
which are high in estrogenic hops, so that wasn't helping.

Low T, even low normal T, may not be optimal. A huge VA study showed that men with their testosterone in the lower normal ranges had more heart problems and earlier death than men in the higher normal T ranges.

So Mark was given testosterone therapy plus an herb to block the testosterone from turning into more estrogen. He was told that the controversy over testosterone being harmful was not accurate.

The controversy about testosterone

There has been a huge controversy about whether or not testosterone therapy is safe in men and whether or not low blood levels of testosterone in otherwise healthy men are dangerous. The emerging science clearly shows that healthy blood levels of testosterone are critical for men, both for their love lives as well as their overall health. While editing this book, almost weekly articles have been coming out that men with higher levels of normal blood testosterone levels have less heart disease, less aggressive prostate cancer if they get it, and even less dementia if they have the Alzheimer's genes. Healthy blood levels of testosterone, not just barely squeaking into the lower range of normal, is critical in keeping men healthy.

Testosterone testing and treating are part of rebooting and maintaining a healthy sex life for many males and females. (There are other causes of low libido besides dysfunctional testosterone signaling). There is a hormone revolution occurring, but since most doctors have not been prescribing hormone therapies for the last decade, you must understand that when you ask many doctors about hormone therapy, be they urologists, gynecologists, endocrinologists, or your general doctors, you have a high probability of getting the wrong answer. I was a keynote speaker in Portland Oregon at a Hormone Boot Camp—a course for relicensing credits for medical doctors, nurse practitioners, naturopathic doctors, and gynecologists. The main message was that too few doctors are truly trained in strategic and safe hormone therapies for both males and females. (Go to http://drlindseyberkson.com/resources for more T info)

Unfortunately, many physicians are still in the dark about the actual science and the benefits. They don't know who can benefit by hormone therapy and who can't, or about the need for maintaining higher normal blood levels for some males, or about how to test and prescribe sanely and safely.

Scary headlines make *louder* news, even with physicians, than headlines that proclaim benefits. This chapter is to set you straight and soothe your concerns surrounding the need and safety of testosterone therapy. Or for you to hand over to the doctor you are asking to test you and potentially balance your testosterone (and other hormone) levels.

Too high or too low

Testosterone signals give men their masculine solidity. And, of course, testosterone is essential for the male libido—the sex drive and urge to connect physically more than emotionally. When testosterone levels are in middle-to-robust ranges, men feel strong and solid and have a sense of reserve and stamina. Excessive levels of testosterone—more than are healthy and necessary—can bring out aggressive traits or an obsession with sex.

As I have said, hormones are all about the Goldilocks principle—the *just right* level. You do not want too-low (insufficient) levels of testosterone or too-high (excessive) levels of testosterone; you want to have the right amount that keeps tissues as healthy as possible. Too many doctors don't understand the concept of *optimal* testosterone levels. They look at the ranges and if you are low normal, they may say your level is sufficient. See? You are still in the normal range even if it is at the near bottom.

· · ·

Hormonal health is all about finding the best levels that work for you, not just the levels that are within the low to high normal blood ranges.

· · ·

But *low end of normal* may not be adequate for *your* personal health. Hormonal health is all about finding the best levels that work for you, not just the levels that are within the low to high normal blood ranges. This concept is crucial to balancing your hormones just right for you! It is prudent to treat you, not just your lab levels!

Optimal levels of testosterone are those that work to give you energy, sex drive, bone health, brain health, and all with the red blood cells staying within normal ranges, too.

Excessively high levels of testosterone aren't good. They have been associated with sudden cardiac death, liver disease, and kidney disease.

Too low levels of testosterone are associated with a large group of factors that aggressively promote heart disease. For example, a study out of England published in the spring of 2016 showed that men with type-2 diabetes who received testosterone replacement had *less* earlier death from *all* kinds of possible causes, especially heart disease. Why? You have been learning that testosterone is a hormone that protects the basic heart cell and health in general. And the brain in particular, in both men and women.

Insufficient levels of testosterone (in normal range, but too low for your ideal health or lower than normal) have been linked with:

- Progression (worsening) of hardening of the arteries (atherosclerosis)

- The production of unhealthy inflammatory molecules, called pro-inflammatory cytokines (testosterone is an anti-inflammatory hormone, especially when mixed with adequate levels of magnesium in your cells and diet)

- Anxiety, depression, and dark moods

- Increased arterial thickness (increases risk of heart disease and high blood pressure)

- Increased levels of glucose (boosts risk of diabetes

- Dementia, memory issues

- Rupture of plaque inside blood vessels, which increases risk of stroke and heart attack), and higher levels of "bad" cholesterols that contribute to dangerous plaque and high blood pressure

- Metabolic syndrome (a number of factors that increase the risks of many illness, including high blood pressure, large belly, high bad fats, low good fats, insulin resistance, and blood sugar issues)

- Less ability to want sex, have sex, and share the sexual experience

- Premature death, especially in those with type-2 diabetes

- More aggressive forms of prostate cancer if you do contract it.

When testosterone levels start to go low

As we grow older, our hormone levels wane. In women, the decrease in estrogen and progesterone occurs fairly abruptly, creating the phase called menopause. In contrast, testosterone levels in men actually start to decline much earlier in life (the start of the *hormonal fall* is around 25 years of age) and continue to go downward slowly over many years, much more slowly than the years before and in menopause in women.

Historically, the decline of male hormones in men, called *andropause*, starts in the early years of adulthood, in the late twenties to the thirties, and then a 1–2 percent reduction per year occurs over a lifetime. This pattern appears to be occurring earlier and escalating.

Approximately 15–25 percent of men over the age of 50 have serum testosterone levels that fall below the threshold considered normal in men between 20 and 40 years old. Yet, clinical reports are coming in that younger men in their twenties and thirties are also becoming deficient in blood levels of testosterone or are non-responsive to whatever levels of testosterone they have! I was at a medical conference in Vegas in 2016. A National of Institute urologist gave a talk about the increasing epidemic of younger men with insufficient testosterone signaling. Obesity, diabetes, eating too much and exercising too little, and environmental pollution are making younger men more feminized and less masculinized.

As you will learn later in the book, a *toxic outer environment* (endocrine damaging chemicals, poor diet, pharmaceuticals, antibiotics, as well as stress and other factors) along with *toxic inner environments* (unhealthy gut bugs, unhealthy gut walls, insufficient nutrients from poor diets, and more) are assaulting our hormones. This includes estrogen, progesterone, thyroid, oxytocin, insulin and others. And, yes, testosterone, too.

Benefits of Testosterone

Testosterone and heart health

When I was a co-lecturer at the American College for the Advancement of Medicine, I heard the famed cardiologist Dr. Stephen Sinatra's riveting lecture. Dr. Sinatra had been a practicing cardiologist for forty years. The first thirty years, he said, he practiced like he had a paper bag over his head. He sent folks for heart replacements and put them on heavy meds and lost a lot of patients to death from heart disease.

Then Dr. Sinatra discovered nutrition and hormone replacement therapy, especially protocols that rebooted the mitochondrial action inside heart cells. Once he knew these protocols, which included testosterone therapy, he could take patients who were set to go to surgery to get a new heart and instead reboot their hearts so thoroughly and rapidly that they didn't need the heart transplant.

Nutrition and hormones help avert transplants—they are that powerful! (Think of what they might do for your sex life.)

T and heart cells

Testosterone signals protect the heart by preventing actual heart cells (cardiomyocytes) from dying *prematurely*. All cells go through normal cycles of birth and death. Cell death, called *apoptosis* (pronounced A-pop-toe-sus) is natural and inevitable. You don't want cells to die too early, especially heart cells. Premature heart cell death puts you are risk of heart attack and early death.

. . .

Testosterone signals protect the heart.

. . .

Researchers from Spain wrote in *Revista Espanola de Cardiologia* in 2010 that testosterone has a *protective* effect on the life cycle of the cardiomyocyte. These researchers showed that *healthy levels* (not very low normal levels) of testosterone deliver signals to cardiomyocytes that keep them younger longer and prevent premature death.

A study published in the *Journal of Clinical Endocrinology & Metabolism* looked at nine observational studies from 1970 to 2013, showing that men with low testosterone levels have a slightly higher risk of developing or dying from heart disease compared to men with higher levels (though still in the normal range). The researchers suggested that too low of testosterone levels could also generate blood clots that might lead to irregular heart rhythms and to more serious heart abnormalities.

In a Swedish study of over 3,000 men with an average age of 75 years, *low* testosterone levels were linked to an increased risk of clogged arteries and heart disease.

One study on men between the ages of 60 and 90 from the First Geriatric Cardiology Department in Beijing, China, found that men with heart disease had lower levels of male hormones and higher levels of female hormones.

Testosterone clearly protects the heart. To walk around with very low normal levels or below normal levels, or with receptors that are damaged and can't take signals from normal levels, all put your heart (not to mention your sex life) at risk.

T and the brain

Both men and women are exposed to increased levels of testosterone through sexual intercourse, and testosterone boosts our brain circuitry. This makes us naturally happier.

Compelling evidence from the psychology department at Florida State University shows that *testosterone protects electrical neural wiring in brains*, which has to do with keeping brains free from anxiety, worry, and depression. One reason women who have had both ovaries removed are more prone to depression, anxiety, and worry is that they now have less testosterone. The ovaries produce much of the testosterone (along with the adrenal glands) in menopausal women. When these testosterone factories are gone, women can get more anxious and depressed.

How does testosterone protect the brain?

One way is that *testosterone protects mitochondria*. These are the energy furnaces deep inside cells that make cells function healthfully. Healthy brains are robust in mitochondria. Unhealthy and aging brains have less.

A new perspective of aging is a *mitochondrial footprint* theory of aging. This way of thinking looks at aging as it is related to loss of these critical energy factories, your mitochondria. This new concept of aging is different from aging as defined as chronological years. Instead, it is looking at the accumulation of oxidative stress that damages and diminishes mitochondrial health.

Healthy testosterone levels protect mitochondria in number and in function, in both Venus and Mars.

Testosterone protects against Alzheimer's disease. There is a gene that puts us at increased risk of developing dementia. But if testosterone levels are at higher but normal blood levels, this gene has less chance to nudge us into cognitive decline. On the other hand, insufficient blood levels of testosterone, together with this gene (ApoE4) are linked to an increased risk of getting Alzheimer's disease.

Research in *The Journal of Alzheimer's Disease* in 2010 studied 153 Chinese men who were at least 55 years or older and didn't yet have dementia. Of these men, 47 had mild cognitive decline, such as problems with clear thinking and memory. Within a year, the ten men who had low testosterone levels as well as high ApoE4 levels went on to develop Alzheimer's disease.

Two brain regions—the hippocampus and cortical regions—have many receptors waiting to receive email messages from testosterone. In fact, the hippocampus has the same order of magnitude of male hormone receptors as the prostate. That's how important testosterone is in the brain. And this holds true for both men and women.

Testosterone is so necessary in the hippocampus, it not only comes in with blood flow from the heart, testosterone is also produced locally right inside the hippocampus. But this local production occurs more in early life and diminishes as we age.

The brain is susceptible to similar damage as the heart. The hallmark of oxidative and inflammatory damage that can assault both the heart and the brain can be *reversed* by testosterone replacement as long as it is given in proper *physiologic* dosages.

A physiologic dose of a hormone is an optimal healthy level that a healthy younger to middle-aged person normally has in their blood.

Testosterone activates a heart protective tool. This has a long name: *extracellular-signal regulated kinases* (ERKs). ERKs block the buildup of nasty oxidative/inflammatory damaging molecules inside cells. ERKs stop damage in both brains, the one in the head and the second brain in the gut (both brains come from the same clump of cells in the fetus and then divide to make the brain in the head and the brain in the gut.) ERKs block nerve breakdown and promotes nerve cell maintenance. And T helps keep this tool humming.

T and cancer

Cancer is thought to occur in three stages—*initiation* (something triggers it), *progression* (it grows), and *metastasis* (it spreads.) Recent science suggests one of testosterone's metabolites, 3 -Adiol, indirectly boosts cancer *protection* by blocking the first of these three dangerous stages. Testosterone thus, in optimal healthy ranges in our bloodstream, helps protect against cancer.

. . .

Men with low levels of the male sex hormone testosterone need not fear that testosterone replacement therapy will increase their risk of prostate cancer.

. . .

Prostate cancer. A study out of New York University's Langone Medical Center and New York University School of Medicine was presented in May 2016 at the annual meeting of the American Urological Association in San Diego, California. In it, they summarized that men with low levels of the male sex hormone testosterone need not fear that testosterone replacement therapy will increase their risk of prostate cancer.

Based on this study, which followed 38,570 men for a number of years to see who got prostate cancer compared to those that did not, and who used T therapy and who didn't, the researchers found T therapy is safe for the prostate.

Concerns have classically come from the fact that standard therapy for advanced prostate cancer uses drugs that drastically reduce rather than increase male hormones. But when T therapy is appropriately used, say these researchers, by men with age-related low testosterone who are otherwise healthy, T replacement has been shown to improve overall health and not raise prostate cancer risk.

These authors highlight that T levels should be kept well within normal ranges to be safe. They wrote that levels below 350 nanograms per deciliter should raise a red flag and that testosterone therapy should be considered (though functional medicine practitioners like to see this level even higher; it depends a lot on how the man feels inside his skin). They even suggest that maintaining normal T levels (avoiding low levels) might protect against exceptional aggressive forms of prostate cancer.

T and cholesterol

Healthy levels of testosterone promote healthier blood fat (lipid) levels. Normal or robust levels of testosterone tend to help cholesterol stay at an optimal level (while too much or too little testosterone does the opposite). Testosterone delivers signals both to the liver and to the lining of blood vessels, which play a role in maintaining healthy levels of cholesterol. Even the conservative Endocrine Society recommends using hormone therapy if blood tests and clinical picture show that men have low testosterone levels because testosterone is heart and cholesterol protective.

T and diabetes

Medical science has shown that men with *low* testosterone have excessive insulin resistance, which is the precursor to type 2 diabetes, obesity, cancer, and even dementia. Increased insulin resistance is also linked to increased body fat, especially abdominal fat and chest fat (man boobs). It is also linked to cognitive decline. Japanese studies on aging men with diabetes show that these men have lower testosterone and higher estrogen levels. Their hormone ratios are opposite what they should be. Pre-diabetes, diabetes, excess weight, and junk food sugary diets are all linked to lower T and higher E (estrogen) levels in men. The lower T levels then worsen these illnesses. It becomes a downward reinforcing spiral. The opposite is also true. Obesity and diabetes can lower testosterone levels. So it can be a two-way nasty street.

Testosterone protects against premature death!

In a scientifically run study with men aged 70 to 96 years old, low testosterone, independent of *any other* preexisting health conditions or risk factors, was associated with an increased risk of dying earlier from any number of causes.

Low blood levels of testosterone levels are linked to an increased risk of *premature death* from heart disease. In a study published in the journal *Heart* in 2010, 930 men who all had coronary artery heart disease were tracked for seven years. Many of these men had low testosterone levels. One out of four men had especially low levels of *free* testosterone, which is the true bioavailable form of testosterone that delivers the actual testosterone signal to the testosterone receptor.

The men were followed for seven years: 41% of the men with low testosterone levels died, compared to 12% of men with normal levels. Deficient levels of *free* testosterone was an independent risk factor for premature death from a wide variety of causes.

Research out of the UK has shown that testosterone replacement in men with type-2 diabetes (on a study of almost 900 males), independently reduced premature death by diverse causes.

It's a mystery to me why people would age and not measure their blood T levels and benefit from better living through modern chemistry if needed.

T and aging

Who wants to get old and saggy with spindly legs? Many issues linked with what has been thought to be inevitable aging in men, including muscle atrophy and weakness, bone loss, reduced sexual functioning, and increased fat mass, especially on the gut and breasts, are similar to changes associated with testosterone deficiency in young men and testosterone deficiency in peri- and post-menopausal women.

These overlaps point to testosterone supplementation as preventing or reversing the effects of aging.

A scientific search was performed to identify studies of testosterone supplementation therapy in older men. In healthy older men with low-normal to mildly decreased testosterone levels, testosterone supplementation increased lean body mass, decreased fat mass, improved bone density, boosted better self-perceived sexual performance, libido, and erectile function. It even caused improvement in men with heart issues, such as exercise-induced coronary ischemia.

T and Erectile Dysfunction

Chicken or the egg? Low levels of testosterone can contribute to erectile dysfunction, but erectile dysfunction can also promote lower levels of testosterone. Things get worse and worse. ED needs to be addressed not just for sexual reasons but also for overall health.

As men live longer, the incidence of erectile dysfunction markedly increases. Men who have *less sexual activity* have lower levels of *free* bioavailable testosterone than men without erectile issues and regular sex lives. (Remember that free testosterone is the form of testosterone that delivers male messages to receptors.)

Erectile dysfunction directly affects men's well-being, self-esteem, inter-personal relationships, and overall quality of life. It is a risk factor for lower testosterone levels and thus more vulnerability to heart and brain issues and disease. So ED is often a canary in the mine, suggesting that these health issues might already be brewing and need to be evaluated. And of course, ED is a basic issue creating a problematic sex life.

Signs of erectile dysfunction include difficulty with:

- getting aroused mentally and physically,
- getting hard,
- sustaining hardness, and
- achieving orgasm.

Clinical trials have demonstrated that testosterone replacement in men that were found *to be low or at the low end of normal* improved overall sexual function and circulation, as well as circulation and health of the penis and associated tissues. T therapy does improve sexual prowess in males that need it.

Benefits of Testosterone for Women

Researchers from the Department of Gynecology and Obstetrics at Faculty Health Science in South Africa reviewed the role of testosterone in women's health. In healthy *post*menopausal women (mature ladies no longer menstruating), the ovaries are supposed to produce significant amounts of androgens (male hormones) for many years after menopause. But women can easily become testosterone deficient. Why?

1. *Age*: Circulating testosterone, like other hormones, decreases with increasing age. Lower levels of testosterone in mature women can cause loss of libido, bone loss, fracture, loss of a sense of well-being, and loss of sensations of sexiness, comfort and pleasure. Notice how many of these symptoms of low testosterone overlap with symptoms we have come to see as inevitable and typical with aging.

2. *Surgery*: Women who have had hysterectomies or who lose both ovaries can have a severe drop in testosterone as ovaries are supposed to be the main source of male hormones in females as we age. But even hysterectomy where ovaries are not removed can lower testosterone. This surgery can sometimes irreversibly affect blood flow to these organs.

3. *Chemicals* in today's environment can reduce testosterone levels in both younger and older women by "clogging" receptors that receive male hormone signals.

4. *Oral estrogen therapy* in postmenopausal women decreases levels of testosterone (by increasing sex hormone–binding globulin, which decreases the body's ability to use the testosterone that is present.) So if your OBGYN puts you on

oral estradiol without testing and treating your testosterone levels, you may be at risk of getting deficient in protective testosterone. And in libido-boosting testosterone!

5. *Antibiotics*: Use of antibiotics can damage the good-to-bad gut bacteria ratio inside our microbiome. When our gut bugs are unhappy, testosterone signals that communicate regularly with gut bugs may not function right. Even if tested levels appear normal! Other medications may do this, too. For example, using acid blocker medications for longer than a month can damage gut bug health and also testosterone functioning.

6. *Too little booty.* Less cuddling and intimacy lowers a woman's T levels.

Testosterone replacement therapy

You can get a script for hormone therapy to replace the testosterone that is lost. Ideally the replacement will be bioidentical, the same form as your body is accustomed to using.

T replacement can help increase muscle mass and bone mineral density and give a sense of solidarity to the otherwise free-fall of emotions that many women experience as they age. I have seen in practice that when midlife women are deficient in testosterone, they are more prone to panic attacks. They have lost the stabilizing hormones they need in their lives. When they are given testosterone replacement, these mood changes and overwhelming feelings often recede, and the patient feels less anxious and more the master of her life.

The more our testosterone levels are optimal, the less overwhelmed and frail we feel. I have had many women who did not feel well with HRT. They complained it "didn't work for them." But their doctors had not added testosterone to the mix. When we did that, then they "felt like a new person."

T protects female hearts

Seventy-five peri- and post-menopausal women were individually tested for estrogens, progesterone, and the male hormones and were given bioidentical hormone replacement for whatever they were deficient or low normal in. Their health was then followed for three years. This is a prospective study, meaning the data is *strong*. There was a "statistically significant" (beyond chance) reduction in inflammatory markers and improvement in heart health markers in women taking hormonal therapies, as well as a better quality of life in spite of high stress reported in most of the women's lives. This was published in the *International Journal of Pharmaceutical Compounding* in January 2013. However, the physician that ran this study lost her academic job at the time because mainstream academia is so antagonistic to bioidentical hormones.

T and depression in women

Anxiety, panic attacks, and depression are some of the top issues that plague middle-aged and aging women. Depression tamps down sexual desire and enjoyment, but so do antidepressants.

Testosterone to the emotional rescue. A trial reported in the *Journal of Sexual Medicine* in 2014 showed that testosterone replacement could reboot libido in women on SSRIs. Forty-four women aged 35 to 55 years, who were on antidepressants and had developed loss of libido due to the drug, were randomly assigned to treatment with a testosterone patch or an identical placebo. The women on testosterone therapy had significant improvement of their libido.

Many women respond favorably to testosterone replacement as a sexual boost in desire and ability to enjoy sex and have an orgasm. This is well documented in the literature and in clinical practice.

It has been reported by researchers, headed by Dr. K. Stephenson from the Women's Wellness Center in Tyler, Texas, that women tested and treated with bioidentical hormone replacement (BHRT) experience *less* depression and could *avoid* antidepressant medication, compared to women not taking HRT. New research is also showing that giving oxytocin replacement can offset the loss of libido in women on SSRI anti-depressants, but may also be able to help women get off the meds themselves.

Testosterone in both men and women is threatened by:

- Not enough sex – *Use it or lose it!* If you're dating and that person, guy or woman, says in their last marriage they had separate rooms, didn't have sex for years if not decades, and at the same times swears to God that they didn't cheat, you can bet their T levels are tanked, their hippocampus is shrunk, and you are getting into a "fixer-upper" big time!

- Too little exercise, especially along with too much sitting. Motion makes more T.

- Hormonally-active pollutants that can hijack testosterone, such as DDT, Bisphenol A, octylpenol, dieldrin, kepone, HPTE, and more. Today's environment is filled with lurking T enemies.

- Exposure to estrogenic pesticides in non-organic foods and from grains and fungus. Eat organic.

- Zinc and other nutrient deficiencies like too little magnesium, along with a junk food diet and poor digestion, impair T signal delivery or cause it to convert to estrogen, effectively lowering testosterone.

- Obesity promotes testosterone conversion into estrogen. Diabetes and obesity can both lower testosterone blood levels, in both men and women, in young males, and even males in their teens if they have enough fat cells to pump out estrogen.

- Excessive alcohol (decreases clearance of estrogen and so raises ratio of estrogen to testosterone).

- Alterations in liver function (decrease clearance of estrogen).

- Aging—increased aromatase activity (promotes conversion of testosterone to estrogen).

- Alterations in gut microbiome (gut bacterial organ of 3-6 pounds that lives inside the intestinal lumen cross-talks with our hormones throughout our lives and, if healthy, helps maintain healthy T levels).

- *Testosterone resistance*—when receptors are clogged with plastics, pesticides, or other chemicals, or nutrient deficiencies block healthy signaling, then signals falter even though blood levels appear normal to your doctor.

- *Too little Vitamin D*—sunshine and Vitamin D help maintain healthy T levels. Inadequate sun exposure, sunscreen and sun exposure through glass can hamper T levels.

Hormone Testing

. . .

When a doctor assesses your hormone levels, ideally he or she should measure all the complete hormone family.

. . .

When a doctor assesses your hormone levels, ideally he or she should measure *all* the complete hormone family: total and free testosterone, DHEA, estradiol, estrone, (estriol in women), progesterone, SHBG, FSH, LH, insulin, TSH, free and total T3, reverse T3, thyroid antibodies, thyroxin-binding globulin, and vitamin D (which is regarded as a *pro-hormone,* meaning it is not only a vitamin but also can act as a hormone).

Testosterone levels regulate lean body mass, muscle size, and strength, while estrogen levels regulate fat accumulation. Sexual performance, including desire and erectile function, are regulated by *both* testosterone and estrogen in *both* men and women.

Exercise and testosterone

Use it or lose it applies to T blood levels.

Research from the Department of Exercise and Sport Science at the University of North Carolina published in 2012 shows that specific forms of exercise can statistically boost *free* levels of bioavailable testosterone. Fifteen males exercised in two different manners, either steady-state endurance or high-intensity interval. *Steady state* is when the exercise effort is pretty stable over the exercise session. *High-intensity* endurance training (a new form that carries a lot of exercise bang for its buck) consists of workouts with *all-out effort* interval bursts for short periods, often 30 to 90 seconds in length. High-intensity intervals are periods when exercisers work out to their utmost levels so that their oxygen use goes up to 110–160 percent of maximal oxygen uptake (VO2 max).

Both forms of exercise boosted testosterone. But get this! The high-intensity interval training appeared to produce a more pronounced use of testosterone by sensitive tissues compared to the regular form of exercise. In other words, high-intensity interval training appeared to make the testosterone more user-friendly to the body (enhanced bio-availability). Cool!

How to increase testosterone levels:

- Enjoy frequent, satisfying sex.

- Exercise (especially with high-intensity intervals as part of your exercise regime).

- If you are taking testosterone and it is converting to estrogen, or your estrogen levels (as a male) are just too high, you can take aromatase inhibitors. They come as pharmaceuticals or natural forms, such as 100 mg grapeseed extract two to three times a day with food. Grapeseed tamps down the gene expression of aromatase enzymes as well as blocking its action, so it doubles as a natural aromatase inhibitor, which keeps T from converting into E.

- Take zinc supplementation (make sure you balance zinc to copper levels, 20 parts zinc to 1 part copper).

- Lose excess weight.

- Don't drink to excess.

- Eat more of the broccoli family foods, which promote healthy processing and removal of excess estrogens.

- Avoid excess grapefruit and pomegranates, as they can inhibit the liver's processing of estrogen if consumed too regularly.

- Take 1–3 g vitamin C daily, which enhances the pituitary gland's responsiveness to changes in hormones and guidance to put things back in balance. In a double-blind randomized controlled trial (top notch science), it was found that taking 3000 mg/day (of time-released vitamin C) boosted sexual frequency in healthy German adults. Higher blood levels of vitamin C were statistically linked to having sex more frequently, and by penile-vaginal style. Of all things, it was not found to boost other styles of sex, like masturbation.

- Take *activated* B complex vitamins to keep hormones balanced.

- Tend to your gut health (microbiome) with digestive enzymes, probiotics, fermented and healthy food choices.

- Bioidentical hormone therapy by prescription.

CHAPTER 7

The Big "O"

Many of my patients complain that they hate to exercise. Wouldn't it be great if you could get stellar health benefits similar to exercising but at the end was an *orgasm?*

Cynthia was 60 years old and had never experienced an orgasm. She admitted this with shame. She had never discussed this with her husband Glen and he had never asked. She described their sex life as tolerable.

Cynthia's main interest was church. Heaven had more "pull" for her than her life on earth, as she looked forward to being reunited with her family. Cynthia also endured severe brain fog.

Upon testing, Cynthia's had no detectable levels of estrogen, testosterone, or any other hormones. The muscles in her arms and thighs were "mushy" on palpation (touch). I reminded her that her heart was a muscle. Her gut, where most of her immune system lived, was lined with muscle. And there were muscles in her pelvis that had to be healthy to be able to contract to achieve an orgasm.

She was started low and slow on hormone replacement and on muscle-building programs for all her muscles, including pelvic. I explained what awakened sex is and how sex is a healthy part of life that helps keep brains younger. I got Glen in and tested his hormones, which were all below normal except his female hormone estrogen, which was high. We discussed how regular, pleasurable, sexual intimacy could keep their cognition more alert and happy. I shared what a G-spot was and how to find it and what this had to do with pleasurable sex.

When Cynthia heard that her brain fog could lift and her desire to be more on earth than in heaven could be rebooted, she was willing to give it a try. Glen ran it by his pastor first, who came in later himself when he heard about their results.

Cynthia called me the morning after her first orgasm. She cried for joy. When she got better at her pelvic exercises, she actually developed the skill to have multiple orgasms. This was a game-changer for their relationship. They became coy, flirty, and vibrant. And of all things, Cynthia felt so much more spry and sharp, she got a job as a receptionist at a local medical hormone clinic where she could encourage potential patients by her own experience. Their satisfied pastor is still sending me patients.

The female orgasm

As we saw in earlier chapters, women are more diverse at the atomic, molecular, and receptor levels. Well, so are their orgasms. But what exactly is a feminine orgasm?

A woman's orgasm is a transient peak sensation of intense pleasure that creates an *altered state of consciousness* for a short time, but a good short time!

Orgasm usually begins with involuntary, rhythmic contractions of the pelvic-vaginal musculature (if her pelvic muscles are out of shape, her orgasms will be, too), often with contractions also in the uterus and anus, with blood buildup in the sexual tissues, followed by a sense of *well-being* and *contentment*. If a woman makes love and fakes an orgasm or does not orgasm, she is not getting this "time out" for her brain and emotions.

Researchers from the Department of Adult Psychiatry at the Medical University of Łód , Poland, investigated the differences between male and female orgasms. These scientists found that in contrast to the male orgasm, the female orgasm is characterized by high *variability* and *diversity*, both in the general population and during one woman's lifetime.

These authors say that women experience sexual pleasure on multiple levels: physical, emotional, spiritual, and intellectual. When a woman orgasms, *all* of her can join in (if she knows how). But emotions, cognitive interpretation of the situation, age, self-esteem, hormone balance, and previous sexual experiences all play a role.

In contrast, according to these scientists, sex for males has more to do with only two factors: arousal and erection. This difference is established by the atoms, molecules, receptors, and rhythm of the male and female hormones, and now we see this echoed in the personality of male and female orgasms.

Mother Nature is consistent!

. . .

The ability to have an orgasm is inherent in males, while in females the ability to have an orgasm has to be acquired by experience and education.

. . .

This data was published in Part 1 of a series. Interestingly enough, in the Part 2 paper, these same researchers state that the ability to have an orgasm is *inherent* in males, while in females the ability to have an orgasm *has to be acquired* by experience and education (like developing a palate for a fine wine). *Sensible sex education is paramount!*

All this research emphasizes the importance of orgasm in a woman as a *complex* process involving the woman's *entire* mind and body. So when making love with women, men should address both the mind and body at the same time, or they are missing part of her sexual boat.

Brain-gasms

The way women experience orgasm has been of interest throughout the ages. But now with the advances of functional imaging techniques, scientists can witness brain activity during orgasm in real time. Women can't fake an orgasm and fool the MRI, so these studies have revealed a whole world happening inside the female brain. Many men would love to have this machine in their homes!

In a study with only females, participants had orgasms while lying under an MRI machine that measured blood flow to different parts of the brain. The Rutgers researchers who led this study, Dr. Barry Komisaruk and Dr. Nan Wise, said that these experiments clearly show that orgasms increase blood flow to *many* parts of the brain in women. The majority of her brain lights up! Brain imaging in males shows that there are fewer brain areas stimulated, making their orgasms less of a "global" brain stimulation and more of a "focused" one.

Brain stimulation from orgasm promotes healthy circulation of blood, nutrients, and oxygen throughout much of the female brain. Thus, when women come, they authentically experience *brain-gasms*. In contrast, mental exercises like crossword puzzles stimulate isolated, specific brain regions. Studies show increased activation in *many* brain regions involved in female orgasm: the paraventricular nucleus of the hypothalamus, in the periaqueductal gray of the midbrain, the hippocampus, and the cerebellum.

Female orgasms turn on a lot of gray matter real estate!

Different types of orgasm

The goal of Dr. R. King and Dr. J. Belsky was to figure out just how many orgasms a woman can experience. A total of 265 females completed an Internet survey and analysis, revealing *two* orgasm types: one on the surface of genitalia, and a second orgasm deeper inside the vaginal vault. The deeper orgasm seems to bring more pleasure and light up more brain areas. (An awakened lover will want to know how to give both types of orgasms to their partner. See chapter 12).

Interestingly, in this study, deeper and more satisfying orgasms had a lot to do with how the woman viewed her partner. Deeper orgasms were associated with partners who were perceived as being more considerate and dominant (manly), with a noticeably attractive smell, and who provided firm penetration. Deeper orgasms that had a sensation of "sucking-in," like the vaginal area is wanting to hold the penis deep inside, along with deep vaginal contractions (which the scientists theorize is the female body wanting to pull in sperm) were found to occur when the woman perceived many positive traits (such as *safety*) about her partner. In this manner, the grabbing-in of the sperm is nature's way of saying, "I want to conceive with this partner."

These same authors later put out another study on 503 women that suggested there were *four* types of female orgasms, two good and two not as good. They concluded that orgasms achieved through masturbation were not as satisfying as those achieved with a partner.

What this research suggests is that orgasms are variable, some deeply satisfying and some more fleeting.

I remember a man I once dated and later became close friends with confiding in me that there is no such thing as a bad orgasm. They were all good. Well, these researchers beg to differ

Clinically, I have known a number of women who, once their hormones are balanced, their nutrition optimized, and both their lovers and vaginas *awakened*, could now enjoy so many orgasms that they lost count. This is the height of sexual pleasure and healthy brain stimulation.

Vaginal orgasm

Awakened sex methods teach women how to have vaginal orgasms with a man. When one learns these easy-to-do steps, you can even do them solo. Maybe if folks knew how to have these while masturbating, there would be more benefits than the research has historically suggested. Most of the negative press about masturbation is that it stimulates a more "clitoral" type of orgasm that mainly affects the "head of the clitoris," but not the middle body and tail. Not a whole hog thing. In my interpretation of the literature, it seems that the *deeper* orgasms are, the more they promote relationship, life, and health benefits.

. . .

Awakened sex methods teach women how to have vaginal orgasms with a man.

. . .

Vaginal orgasm can be learned, like anything else, through due diligence. Practice-makes-perfect. One study showed that the more a woman could be taught to focus her attention on vaginal sensations during lovemaking, the more often a woman could achieve vaginal orgasm. In this study, where women made love with male partners, women did find that vaginal orgasms were easier to achieve if the penis was longer and harder. In regard to vaginal orgasms, *size* can matter. But *talent* can override size issues! And that comes with *education*.

Non-genital orgasm

There is proof that orgasm can be achieved without actually stimulating the genitalia. It's not too common though. Drs. Komisaruk and Whipple suggest that genital orgasm is a special case of stimulation of clitoral tissue but that orgasm can occur from other areas of the body being touched, and even without physical touch anywhere on the body if enough emotionality and mutuality is happening!

These same authors wrote that love is so critical it is like air and food. People who do not have intimacy in their lives may be more vulnerable to psychosomatic illness (physical un-wellness secondary to emotional un-wellness) as they are less exposed to the *natural healing force that making love generates*. This scientific article suggested that.

Prolactin: The "ah" hormone of sexual satisfaction

In women, sexual *frequency* is not the golden ring as much as sexual *satisfaction*. Scientific studies, like the Women's Health Observational Sex

Study, demonstrate that. If a woman could look back over her sexual life history and feel a sense of fulfillment, pleasure, and love—well, that's the Holy Grail. She lives longer and with a greater sense of well-being compared to women who perceive their sexual history as unsatisfying and unfulfilling.

. . .

In women, sexual frequency is not the golden ring as much as sexual satisfaction.

. . .

Remember, her hormones and receptors are diverse and complex. A woman needs a *lot more to take place within the sexual arena* to have a satisfying whole mind and body experience than a man does. This may not hold true for all men and women, but it does for most.

Not all orgasms are equal. Some give more pleasure than others. It depends on how much of the satisfaction hormone, prolactin, your brain releases. Part of having an amazing orgasm is based on how much prolactin the experience got your brain to produce.

Dr. S. Brody, along with Dr. T.H.C. Kruger, ran three studies comparing how much of *prolactin* a brain produced depending on how the orgasm was experienced. These studies were performed in laboratories, where men and women either masturbated or engaged in regular penile-vaginal intercourse. At the moment of orgasm, their blood levels of prolactin were immediately measured.

There was a *400 percent greater* prolactin release following intercourse with a mate than following masturbation. The authors say that intercourse is more *physiologically satisfying* than masturbation. And more brain stimulating.

Brain stimulation comparing love combinations:

- *Best*—making love with a beloved in which the situation is "safe" and "appropriate" enough to not use a condom.

- *Next best*—making love with a great lover who can turn you on even though you are not over the moon in love.

- *Least*—love the one you're with; still get some bennies from solo masturbation but down on the totem pole.

· · ·

There was a 400 percent greater prolactin release following intercourse with a mate than following masturbation.

· · ·

If you are just putting up with sex for your mate's sake, or doing it because the TV is broken, or you are engaging in intimacy with a friend with benefits, or by yourself at night under your lonesome sheets, then you are having legitimate but less satisfying sex, as far as your brain and total body health are concerned.

Masturbation

With masturbation, you still get relief, you still get to orgasm, but you make less oxytocin, get less boost of whole body circulation, less brain-gasmic benefits, and some of the literature even suggests there are some shadow sides to solo sex.

Some research shows that masturbation frequency (and even just the desire to do so) has been associated with depression and inversely associated with love! The more you masturbate, the less love you have in your life. Well, maybe that makes sense. The more you are not in a relationship, the more you are going to sexually "take care of yourself." I theorize the depression came first and the social isolation and masturbation came next. It is not necessarily the other way around.

However, my opinion aside (since I am presently single), masturbation is repeatedly shown in the peer review scientific literature to be inversely associated with good mental health when this style of sex is compared to other types of partnered sex. In other words, more sex by yourself, less happiness.

I think there are two possible explanations not addressed in theses studies.

1. It might that through masturbation we develop a better sense of how to please ourselves exactly right. If you do not tell your partner what you learned in private, how can your partner help you achieve the highest pleasure? What pleasure you get with another might fail by comparison. So share what you learn by masturbation with your lover. This knowledge promotes better pleasure and happier relationships between the two of you.

2. The more alone we are, the more we would have solo sex, since that is the present "is-ness" of a single person's situation. And there are lots of singles. The United States, for the first time in history, had slightly more than half of its adult population (according to census taking) now in single-dom. Does this mean that all single people who masturbate are depressed or need more scripts for anti-depressants? *No!* But it does mean that if we are not in a relationship, we have to find other things to be happily "relational toward"—such as community, friends, work, and workers we connect with—or else we can easily fall prey to depression.

There is no perfect way to be single or in a relationship. Many people, as I learn from speaking with my patients, are in relationships but at the same time are sad and lonely. So we are talking about maximizing human happiness and health, no matter what life has dealt you.

It does not mean that if we are single, or our husband is overseas, or paralyzed, or whatever our unique fate, that we should not masturbate or that clitoral climax is never good unless we are coming simultaneously. The science suggests that some people who masturbate may be more prone to social and emotional isolation. But if you are solo and masturbate, and yet have strived to achieve a dynamic community life, this may not apply to you.

I have always thought it is better to release oneself than to not do so. I do not think that the negative masturbation studies mean that you shouldn't masturbate to release tension, stimulate blood flow, or have some personal enjoyment with no muss or fuss. But the studies do emphasize that we appear to be set up at a neurobiologic level to enjoy sex with a regular partner. Or learn how to have brain-gasmic, multiple, deep orgasms on our own!

Do women ejaculate?

When women make love, sometimes fluids are squirted out like a mini-version of the male ejaculation. This is called *female ejaculation*, which has been discussed and robustly debated for over 2,000 years. What are these fluids? Are they an ejaculate like men produce? Some studies say women are just experiencing release of urine that builds up in the bladder during sex. Other studies say that women do in fact ejaculate and that this ejaculate is different from diluted urine and is, when analyzed, similar to components of male semen.

Dr. Rubio-Casillas and Dr. E. A. Jannini presented a case report in the *Journal of Sexual Medicine* providing biochemical proof of release of an authentic female ejaculate that is expressed along with some diluted urine. They concluded that the ejaculation that some women do, and squirting and gushing and dripping that most women do, are two different phenomena. They even demonstrated a bona fide difference between the organs and the mechanisms that produce these fluids. These researchers were detail oriented. They said that the true female ejaculation is the release of a very scanty, thick, and whitish fluid from the female prostate, (the female Skene's glands and ducts), while the squirting is the expulsion of a diluted fluid/urine from the bladder.

Other scientists, Drs. F. Wimpissinger, C. Springer, and W. Stackle also wanted to know if women could ejaculate. Their research demonstrated that female ejaculate typically consists of about two ounces of a specific ejaculation fluid. They said their research proves this feminine ejaculate is not vaginal secretions (vaginal transudate) or plain old urine. They say, yes, some ladies do, like men, ejaculate fluid.

118

Research suggests that about half of all women actually ejaculate during sexual stimulation. An online questionnaire assessed data from 320 women who claimed they ejaculated regularly, and the scientists followed these women's sexual reporting of their experiences for one-and-a-half years. The woman all said they ejaculated exactly at the time of orgasm. About 80 percent of the women and 90 percent of their partners perceived female ejaculation as a good thing and an enrichment of their sexual lives.

However, there is a definite lack of consensus on the matter. One study reported that it is more unusual to find women that ejaculate (10 to 54 percent of women reported ejaculating in this study) and that it is more often urinary incontinence caused by penile penetration rather than true ejaculation. Another study by the Department of Obstetrics and Gynecology from Hôpital Privé de Parly 2, in France, says there is no female ejaculate. They have measured it and they say it's merely urine.

In the science of female sex, there is a huge lack of agreement. The sexual science around men is more congruent. Why? Women are more complex and men are simpler, so you just gotta laugh.

In my practice, women frequently report to me that when they become more comfortable with sex, when their hormones are balanced either naturally (herbs, foods, and nutrients) or with replacement, when they practice *awakened* sex and look at their mate with the new understanding of how we are hardwired at the deeper level of sex hormones, and start to enjoy deeper or multiple orgasms, they naturally start to ejaculate even when they never did that before!

And yes, grateful patients report the ability of women to ejaculate does seem to intensify the orgasmic experience for both partners!

Awakened sex

What does it mean when a woman is "awakened?" It means she is awakened to the difference between men and women from the atoms up; it means that her hormones are balanced so her tissues are awakened with health; it means that she and her lover approach sex with the intention to be more connected so that they both get to experience more pleasure and their brains are more turned on; it means that they know where and how to touch and speak with each other based on their atoms and their brains—and the whole experience is bigger and more complete and more satisfying. This is *awakened sex*.

. . .

*Awakened sex is bigger and more complete
and more satisfying.*

. . .

The more a woman has heightened sex, the more pleasure the man has, too. Men love to be respected and appreciated and they take a moaning happy woman as an appreciative woman. They have been the rock. They have anchored her emotionality and ups and downs with their ability to deliver amazing pleasure. When a woman receives great pleasure and lets the man know it, it is very giving to a man. And very satisfying to him, too.

If a woman has not had the experience of awakened sex, if she has not had mind-boggling orgasms, nor felt deeply connected and held and appreciated while making love, then most likely she is going to be a woman who is not very interested in regular, frequent lovemaking. It behooves a man and woman to give each other deep pleasure so they both keep wanting to come together and, in doing so, promote the health and happiness of each other. And ultimately, their entire family if they have one. Happier parents make for happier families.

According to scientific literature, it is clear that emotionality, which science often refers to as the *emotional field*, plays a greater role in sexuality and orgasmic ability with most women than with most men. Even if a man isn't in love with a woman, if he approaches making love with her by awakened steps, which mean by bonding on a number of levels through touch, words, and connection, and addressing her body and mind by how she is wired in her atoms, this should heighten her experience, which should then heighten his. This is the *hormone love language*. This name is very accurate indeed.

120

Sex should be the ultimate win-win. The ultimate give and give and give and take. Too often it is just a take. And then, of course, who wouldn't have a headache?

Come together

There is research that looks at the benefits of coming (orgasming) together. One study was done on 1,570 Czechs and the information was gathered through surveys. The authors, out of University of West of Scotland, School of Social Sciences, Paisley, UK, headed by none other than Dr. S. Brody, concluded that penile-vaginal frequency and *simultaneous orgasm* made each man and woman achieve the happiest of all states of sexual interactions.

One of the reasons I am writing about awakened brain-gasmic sex is that when men and women get taught how and why to come together, their lives get better on all levels. Young couples will want to be educated with step-by-step information and be able to go about it without guilt. Moms will want their sons and daughters to know this information so they can achieve healthier marriages and avoid divorce.

Many admit to me in the privacy of our clinical interaction that their religious teachings made them feel guilty about sex, or their parents made them feel badly about sex. They have no idea how to go about it, or why they should get guilt-free pleasure from it. The 2015 study out of Sweden found that one out of three Swedish couples are separating before one of their kids is five years old, partially due to lack of sensuality, sexuality, and connection. The scientists offered tips to save Swedish marriages. One tip was learning how to be better lovers. And how to insert *sensuality* into daily life.

Nature gave us orgasms to keep us connected. Orgasms make our brains produce connecting hormones. We can be better connected with life, with ourselves, our children and with God, who created this marvelous body and the ability to orgasm. We become happier parents able to create a happier home. Nature is all tending the next generation.

. . .

Nature gave us orgasms to keep us connected.

. . .

Learning how to get out of our heads and into the rest of our body and connect (be it with another person or other parts of ourselves) creates the terrain for us to receive all that nature makes possible with the *gift of orgasm*. (Go to http://drlindseyberkson.com/resources for more on oxytocin)

CHAPTER 8

Oxytocin—The Multi-Tasking Cuddle Chemical

*W*hen Sheila walked into my office, I was struck by how attractive she was—a slim, long-legged, dark haired knockout. But something was wrong.

Sheila grabbed the Kleenex, dabbed her teary eyes and explained. She had a 16-year old daughter that she loved but didn't love. She had a husband she loved yet didn't love. She cared for them but had no desire to touch, interact, or be close to them.

It started during pregnancy with her daughter. Early in the first trimester she had what seemed like a mini stroke. The ER couldn't find anything wrong. For 48 hours, one side of her was numb and difficult to move. It left as mysteriously as it had occurred.

After that Sheila shuffled through life. When her daughter was born she didn't feel what she thought other moms felt. She no longer wanted to make love or hang with her girlfriends. She begged for a hormonal fix.

I had just ended my first year of working and studying with an internist and hormone specialist in Tulsa, OK, who had been using oxytocin replacement for several year, in both men and women to enhance intimacy. I learned how and when to use it.

Sheila left the office with a prescription in hand.

She returned one month later. She reported that after several days on the oxytocin therapy she felt like hugging and hanging with her daughter. She felt like making love with her husband again. She could "connect."

That's oxytocin.

Successful sex is successful connection. If you go on the Internet and read dating profiles, 90% of them say they are looking for *connection*. Most of us long to connect. Well, there is a hormone of connection, called *oxytocin*.

During sex, through the build-up of energy and release with orgasm, oxytocin is produced and secreted into the brain and bloodstream. When oxytocin delivers its messages to the brain, anatomical areas linked with *connection, bonding,* and *empathy* are lit up. Oxytocin boosts special perceptions between partners, like making the one with whom you are orgasming appear more attractive to you.

Oxytocin is part of nature's plan to "woo" us to stay together for the benefit of the family and the next generation.

How oxytocin accomplishes connection

Animal research first figured out how oxytocin does its attachment magic and just how powerful it is. These investigations began with a small mouse-type rodent called the vole.

Two closely-related species of voles have two opposite relationship styles. One vole is monogamous, mating for life. The other species of vole is promiscuous, choosing to be a forever player. What's the biological difference? The monogamous vole has much more oxytocin activity in the brain. In comparison, the polygamous vole has much less.

Researchers wanted to see just exactly how powerful a pull oxytocin has on mating choices. They altered the numbers of oxytocin genes and thus oxytocin signaling. By reducing or increasing oxytocin signals in the brain, they could reproducibly switch the mating habits of the voles. They could morph the player vole into a monogamous vole. And vice versa. By turning on more or less oxytocin signaling, they could create biologic monogamy or bigamy (or should we say "pig-amy").

Other researchers "gene jerry-rigged" oxytocin even more. They could, by manipulating oxytocin in the animal's brain, drive an animal to choose a specific mate over others. This is rather mind boggling to the gray matter. It's now theorized that this is what men and women do. That part of our choice of partners and staying with them is somewhat a result of our brain hormones.

It's clear. Oxytocin deserves to be called "the cuddle hormone," "the love hormone," and "the cuddle chemical."

What exactly is oxytocin?

Oxytocin is a *peptide hormone*, meaning it is made from proteins. This is different than estrogen and testosterone, which are sex steroid hormones. There are two basic types of hormones: steroid and peptide. Both have to bind to a receptor, but they bind to different types of receptors.

However, oxytocin is more than just a hormone. It is also a *neurotransmitter*. So oxytocin is both a hormone and a neuropeptide. This means that it has hormonal activity like hormones do, but it affects brain tissue like neurotransmitters do, especially in *both* our brains (in our head and in our gut).

Oxytocin is made throughout the day in both the male and female brain, in small pulsing amounts. It's made in the hypothalamus (inside the brain) and delivered to the pituitary (inside the brain), which secretes it through its backside, called the posterior pituitary, into the bloodstream to travel all over the body. It delivers signals to tissues that have oxytocin receptors, the hormonal satellite dishes that receive oxytocin signals. Many tissues have oxytocin receptors. For example, your gut and muscles need oxytocin signals to stay healthy and strong.

Oxytocin has historically been thought of as a pregnancy and breast-feeding hormone. During labor and breastfeeding, natural oxytocin from the mother (not to be confused with oxytocin replacement) flushes both the mom and baby's body. In this way, mother's oxytocin is yet another way nature helps trigger a healthy baby microbiome and intestinal tract. We have long known that vaginal delivery helps "seed" the baby's microbiome (I wrote about it in *Healthy Digestion the Natural Way* and *Natural Answers for Women's Health*) but so does the natural flushing of the infant's system with oxytocin hormone gifted to them by their mother's bloodstream!

So oxytocin is an integral part of giving birth and the bonding of mother to child during breastfeeding. But we are learning that it is much more—all the way from maintaining a healthy gut, avoiding leaky gut, preserving muscle so that it ages more slowly, to helping maintain healthy weight, to boosting sexual desire and capability. And orgasm strength!

Oxytocin is being looked at to treat not only intimacy and connection issues, but also to treat digestive woes like leaky gut, and anxiety issues from fight-or-flight stressed out nervous systems.

Oxytocin is a Buddha-like hormone. It calms tissues. It's a healer. A bonder. A connector of the dots to keep us Zen-like. That's why we feel so relaxed after the big "O." Our brains are flush with oxytocin. In fact, meditation partially provides some of its benefits by boosting the production of oxytocin.

Oxytocin and orgasms

When you orgasm, the pituitary secretes oxytocin and prolactin. These hormones circulate in the brain and then through the body. When oxytocin and prolactin signal the brain, you feel warm and connected with your lover. When the bloodstream carries the oxytocin to the pelvic regions, it promotes vaginal and uterine movements as well as enhancement of sperm and egg transport. But as we find out about non-sexual organs having oxytocin receptors, we learn more about its health-boosting benefits throughout our bodies. Especially with regular intimacy.

. . .

You can't fool Mother Nature.

. . .

It turns out that only *actual* orgasm gives the biggest boost of pituitary blood flow, and thus enhances the greatest secretion of oxytocin and prolactin. You can't fool Mother Nature. If a woman is touched on her clitoris or other parts of her body, or even if a man enters her, but she does *not* have a real orgasm, if she fakes an orgasm, her pituitary will still not squirt out extra oxytocin or prolactin.

As lovemaking builds, as tension mounts, with each phase of sex for both the woman and the man, the level of oxytocin rises in the bloodstream. Why? To boost connection. Between each person. Between the egg and the sperm. But it's with orgasm that the largest amount of oxytocin is produced.

Immediately after orgasm, oxytocin levels rise significantly in the brain and bloodstream in both men and women. They remain exceedingly elevated for only about five minutes. Then levels rapidly decline.

- Sex between men and women *without* coming to an orgasm makes less oxytocin.

- Faked orgasms can't fake the pituitary.

- Orgasms by clitoral manipulation, between men and women, produces even less.

- Solo orgasms achieved by masturbation boost less secretion of oxytocin and prolactin than "shared" orgasms.

Gender-bending oxytocin

Oxytocin is an orgasm hormone, and the more connected you are, the more you make. But it is the female brain that produces the most oxytocin. Much more than the male brain.

During orgasm (proven by PET-neuroimaging), the pituitary gland is turned on, more so in the female brain than the male. So when a woman screams out "O God," she gets more of a healthy thunderbolt to her pituitary. The pituitary is considered the body's master gland, located in the middle of the brain. It is so much the ultimate director of what goes on inside the body that the pituitary actually has a higher blood flow going to and through it than all other parts of the brain or body (except for the *carotid body* in the neck that dumps directly into the pituitary).

In a study with 11 healthy women, orgasm instantly increased the blood supply and flow rate right into the pituitary gland. *Orgasms thus turn the pituitary on.* More blood flow to the pituitary boosts more production of oxytocin and prolactin—the love hormone and the satisfaction hormone—creating feelings of *connection* and *pleasure*.

Since the female brain secretes more oxytocin and prolactin than the male brain, when she orgasms, she *longs* to *bond* and has tremendous *satisfaction* with that sensation.

. . .

The female brain is built to bond and hard-wired
to remember how female has always needed male.

. . .

No matter how much a "friend with benefits" male lover might insist a liaison is only a friendly wham bam, thank you ma'am, if it's done often enough, and she orgasms enough, she'll bond with him. Her brain and hormones make her do it.

If the man's emotions come along with the sex, he can be open to bonding, but he mentally has to choose to do so. If he is not into you,

128

multiple orgasms do not turn on his brain to want to bond with you no matter how many regular trysts you share.

Oxytocin is not just about orgasms

Since there are oxytocin receptors all over your body, oxytocin signals many tissues other than the brain and genitals. This shows how love making can gently boost health in so many cells, not just reproductive and brain cells. Body tissues, other than the brain and pituitary, that contain significant oxytocin receptors are:

- Thymus

- Heart

- Pancreatic islet cells (the cells that make insulin, so oxytocin therapy is being looked at to prevent and perhaps treat diabetes)

- Kidney (oxytocin is being looked at to protect against chronic kidney decline, especially in diabetics)

- Ovary (female sexual organ)

- Testes (male sexual organ)

- Vascular epithelium (lining of blood vessels so oxytocin therapy is being looked at for heart health support)

- Adipocytes (oxytocin is being looked at for appetite reduction and weight loss)

- Osteoclasts/ osteoblasts (oxytocin is being looked at to protect bones!)

- Myoblasts (oxytocin protects muscles from aging and also may help some pain and fibromyalgia patients, though the results are conflicting)

- Several types of cancer cells (oxytocin may help your immune system fight certain cancer cells)

- Gut and vagus nerve (oxytocin helps prevent and treat inflammation in the gut and leaky gut, and helps a gut become more parasympathetic (calmer and digestively healthy)

The brain is flush with oxytocin receptors. So is the vagus nerve, which is the next largest network of nerves second only to the spinal chord. The vagus nerve is our electrical input into our calming, parasympathetic nervous system (the opposite of the fight or flight sympathetic one). Inside the brain and inside the vagus nerve is a hotbed of oxytocin receptors. The brain and our calming nervous system long to get emails from oxytocin telling these structures to chill out. To keep their heads.

Exactly next to these receptors are an almost twin set of receptors, they are so close in location. These are the estrogen beta receptors. In both males and females. If you remember, these are the satellite dish receptors that receive signals protecting *against* cancer.

This twosome team, oxytocin and estrogen receptor beta signals, work in cozy consort to help the body fight cancer. And for tissues to achieve physiologically Zen-ness and health!

Oxytocin therapy is a hotbed of interest for diverse clinical applications. A fascinating factoid is that oxytocin is increased the more we go through emotionally difficult times. It's one way hardship helps us to develop empathy. In other words, this hormone helps us learn from emotional crisis.

If your husband or wife is flat-lined, non-responsive, and aggravatingly non-empathetic, perhaps the right dosage and timing of oxytocin therapy would turn their compassion back on. Remember, hormones dictate how we see the world, how we interact in the world, and how we attempt to treat and love each other. Hormone replacement can be used to treat, balance, and promote better health in all of these arenas.

But remember, all things in biology are individual. Each person secretes dissimilar amounts of hormones from similar experiences. I may produce more oxytocin when I orgasm than you, or vice versa. And we each respond uniquely to persons, places, and timing. We all have our own hormonal footprints. Or in this case, *orgasm footprints*. Or perhaps, *compassion footprints*.

Honeymooners make the most oxytocin—strategic nature once again.

Women produce more oxytocin upon orgasming, which makes women want to connect and nest. But at the beginning of a relationship, in the *bonding period*, both the man and the woman make more oxytocin. When men are more willing to be open, they start to produce less testosterone during this transient time. This hormonal symphony— more oxytocin opening their bonded-ness, more testosterone in the woman from all the cuddling, and less testosterone in the man from all his openness—sets the hormonal scene for the heart merge that connects their "emotional" hearts together physiologically.

The more intense the bonding, the more their brains (being an explosion of connecting oxytocin) are glued together in love. The longer couples participate in the honeymoon period, including hot sexual interactions, gazing into each other's eyes, and intense periods of quality time together, the more both their brains become booming oxytocin factories. This *oxytocin-fest* (along with male lower T and female higher T) becomes the stick-together-ness of a healthy relationship that helps the couple weather bad times when they show up down the road (which, of course, they eventually do for all of us).

Thus, the honeymoon period is nature's way to protect the next generation by building a bridge for this relationship from the present through to the future.

The eight-year Gothenberg study in Sweden, which looked at how to keep Swedish couples from breaking up their families, recommended the 3 C's to keep couples happy and families stable: *commitment, cuddling,* and *chemistry*. If couples could be sensual in and out of the bedroom, if they could learn how to connect, the chemistry generated kept families together. These are all actions of oxytocin, whether it is produced by orgasm or given as a prescription!

The power of oxytocin (connection) is real.

Men and oxytocin

Oxytocin is not only an orgasm hormone. The male brain produces very small amounts of oxytocin about every half hour all day long. Comparative PET-scan studies show that during orgasm, men's pituitaries don't get as large boosts of blood flow and thus are not as turned on as women's. So their orgasm burst of oxytocin is less than what a female brain produces. In fact, some men have no pituitary activation with orgasm at all. So males, at time of orgasm, produce lower levels of oxytocin and prolactin compared to women.

I'm sure you've heard about Viagra. Well, it partly works by boosting oxytocin production in males. Researchers at the University of Wisconsin-Madison demonstrated that rat pituitaries treated with Viagra (chemical name Sildenafil) secreted three times more oxytocin upon stimulation compared to control mice not getting the medication. So Viagra's actions are partially due to boosting the body's production of oxytocin.

Another study measured blood levels of oxytocin at the time of orgasm in both men and women, who indicated the start and finish of the orgasm by pushing a button. Yes, both men and women made oxytocin at time of orgasm. But women made more and men made less.

If a man gives a woman mind-boggling orgasms and makes love with her regularly, and is then ruffled by her feeling bonded to him even though he may have "warned" her that he wasn't interested in marriage or monogamy, he is going against her physiologic reality.

Some men find that testosterone replacement *combined with oxytocin* increases their ability to enjoy, as well as bond, during sexual interaction.

Oxytocin to the rescue

I had a patient, a surgeon, who was a very fit senior in a new relationship with a man many decades younger. She admitted she loved sex but, even after several husbands, she had never experienced a real orgasm.

She had been on estrogen, progesterone, and testosterone replacement for years, which was helping other things, but not this. She had libido, but no follow-through.

I recommended oxytocin.

I got a message from her several days later. She reported that she made love all night and couldn't stop orgasming. It was the best sex ever for both of them. No more faking for her!

That's oxytocin.

Oxytocin replacement

If for some reason your body is not making oxytocin in the amounts that your tissues want or require, then replacement with it can be like magic. But if your levels are not low or that is not your physiologic "weakest link" issue, then taking oxytocin, no matter the dose or delivery mode, may not feel like it is making much difference for you. It is not a miracle answer for everyone.

But since so many tissues have oxytocin receptors, you may be receiving *silent* benefits. For example, it may preserve muscle or it may help silently heal a leaky gut wall (an intestinal lining that is not guarding against the wrong things from inside the gut getting into your blood stream).

- *Dosage is everything.*
- As well as timing.
- As well as how you take it inside your body called delivery mode.

Most of the research uses a nasal spray (called intranasal spray) or gels made for application inside the vagina.

Oxytocin replacement is well tolerated, and appears to have no adverse effects other than it does not work for everyone across the board. It may help lower excessively high stress (cortisol) hormone blood levels,.

People with severe adrenal fatigue already have too little cortisol, so they may have to try oxytocin therapy slowly, if at all.

The Hormone Health Network (lay audience arm of the Endocrine Society) states that too high oxytocin levels can cause benign enlargement of the prostate, but investigation by a top oxytocin researcher (Dr. Michael Kaplan from Tahoma Clinic in Tukwila, WA) says that this cannot be substantiated and, in fact, appears to be the opposite.

Theoretically, if you take too much oxytocin, you may get "sticky dependent behaviors" and be overly sensitive to behavioral or facial cues, but this would cease by reducing the dose. I don't know of studies that have tested this and I have not seen this in patients.

Oxytocin increases men's desire to "share"

In a study published in the *International Journal of Psychology*, 60 adult men were asked questions about their various personal characteristics. They were then given a placebo or oxytocin and had to watch a movie featuring friendship and camaraderie. Then they were asked to recall a past negative experience *that currently affected them* and rate its emotional intensity at the time. Participants had to indicate whether they would agree to share the related facts and emotions with another person.

Analysis of the results showed that *oxytocin increased the willingness of men to share their emotions.* The authors called the findings remarkable. Remember, hormones dictate how we experience our personal "reality show."

Oxytocin as pain reliever

Dr. Jorge D. Flechas was the first to introduce oxytocin to the medical community around the 1970s. He did this in relation to using it to treat patients with fibromyalgia—a chronic condition in which the patient suffers with severe chronic fatigue and pain, but is often unresponsive to conventional meds. Dr. Flechas became aware of the application of oxytocin to reduce pain and increase well-being and energy in these patients when one of his severely ill clients reported that she only experienced pain relief during and for a short time after orgasm.

An old scientific article discussed how sex could reduce pain for up to six hours in some patients with rheumatoid arthritis. How? Probably by boosting oxytocin levels, which act to reduce pain.

I had a patient with severe chronic vestibulolopathy—chronic brain inflammation that manifests with dizziness, nausea, and fatigue. None of the really smart docs she had seen were able to help her. She reported to me that the only time she felt well was right after orgasm. She is finding some relief with oxytocin therapy. It isn't making her problem go completely away but it is better than any of the other expensive treatments she has tried over the last three years.

Better sex up your nose?

Dr. A. Burri and colleagues ran a study in 2008 where they gave intranasal oxytocin to ten patients and had them each go on to orgasm. The participants went through this test twice, once on the oxytocin and the next time on placebo. They were asked to identify which time they were given the oxytocin or the placebo.

Eight out of ten subjects correctly perceived when they had indeed been given oxytocin.

Why? All ten said they had a better experience of sex and orgasm when on the oxytocin. And eight out of ten could say "on the money" when this arousal was due to oxytocin. It was a small study, but it pointed to oxytocin enhancing the experience of intimacy.

Dr. B. Behnia and co-workers ran a randomized controlled study on 29 heterosexual couples They were given nasal sprays, either placebo or a nasal dose of 24 IU of oxytocin (this is the common dosage used in many human trials). After sex, they filled out surveys.

Men felt more satisfied after sex. Women felt more relaxed. But the men responded more powerfully to the therapy than the ladies, feeling much more empathetic as they felt their hearts opened up more! Perhaps because women already produce more oxytocin than men, men may be set up to be more responsive to it.

Oxytocin for ED (erectile dysfunction).

If a man has trouble orgasming it is called *anorgasmia*.

The first discussion about using oxytocin for ED in the scientific literature was by Dr. W. W. Ishak, who had an 82-year-old gent that nothing else had helped. You might think, hey, he's 82, give up the ghost. But he has a right to a great sex life. Wait till you are 82!

By using oxytocin nasal spray, the patient was able to achieve multiple orgasms per week. The patient was happy and the benefits continued as long as he used the oxytocin spray.

Oxytocin exerts influence in the central nervous system and in the peripheral by stimulating the release of nitric oxide. This molecule, nitric oxide, can metaphorically be dubbed the "yoga molecule" as it makes blood vessels relax and open wider, healthfully boosting circulation. This is how many of the erectile dysfunction drugs do what they do, by boosting nitric oxide and improving blood flow into the penis in a man and the clitoris in a woman. Oxytocin has similar actions.

Oxytocin face lift?

What if you could make your lover see you as more attractive, even without a face lift? Oxytocin replacement was given to 20 couples in a randomized fashion. Some got placebo, some got oxytocin, but all got their brains scanned with MRI imaging. After sex, men were shown photos of the woman they had just been with, and how they scored the attractiveness of the ladies they had just made love with was recorded. When male noses were sprayed with oxytocin, they felt the women they made love with were, hands down, more attractive than ladies they had not made love with.

Now, what did the look-see with MRIs show inside the brain? As oxytocin entered the brain through the olfactory bulb (by being sprayed into the nasal passageways), the part of the brain lit up that turns on a man's *appreciation of attractiveness*. It did this for photos of his partner but not for unfamiliar women or even other women he did know.

- Oxytocin turned the male's brain on to his female.

- Oxytocin turns on an area in a man's brain where he "sees" you as someone he wants to be with above all others.

- It ups the probability for him to want to stay with you.

The authors say that their results suggest that oxytocin helps with the romantic bond between man and woman.

I wonder . . .

When we make love with someone regularly, nature gifts us connection and turns on our brain to make us "see" this person as attractive Then we are driven to have more sex. And then we bond even more. It's a positive feedback loop. The more the baby suckles, the more oxytocin is released; the more milk lets down, the more the baby suckles. The more you make love, the more you bond and the better you look to each other. That is what the early stage of a relationship is. And with awakened sex practices, you can create this on an ongoing basis even after the honeymoon is over. This makes for a happier couple that is more likely to stay together. Oxytocin gets you so bonded through your brain and mutual sex that you do whatever it takes to make your relationship work.

• • •

Nature uses oxytocin as a sex therapist.

• • •

Nature uses oxytocin as a sex therapist; we learn to long to stay and for it all to work out for our highest good. Nature gives us pleasure, wants

137

love to stay, and the family to be safe. Oxytocin turns on your brain to protect the next generation and to love the one you're with.

Oxytocin and SSRI medications

Millions of people are depressed and take SSRI drugs to treat depression by boosting serotonin. But these drugs lower oxytocin, which is inhibited by serotonin. This is one reason that antidepressants can lower sexual drive and ability.

In a rodent study, males were chemically made unable to orgasm. Dr. T.R. De Jong and his team showed that oxytocin administration reversed this impairment.

Taking oxytocin replacement while taking SSRI antidepressants can reverse this very depressing and damaging sexual side effect. If you are on SSRI meds and have trouble making love, try oxytocin.

Oxytocin for high risk women

Many women cannot or do not want to take estrogen. They have had breast cancer or they don't like hormones. Well, oxytocin to the rescue. Oxytocin taken as a vaginal gel acts on the vagina like estrogen, without ANY estrogenic activity.

A pilot study was run on 20 post-menopausal women with atrophic vaginitis. This is when the vaginal walls get dry and thin and a woman finds making love painful, and she might even bleed. The women were given oxytocin gel or a placebo gel.

Once a day they placed some gel into their vaginas. After seven days, seven out of ten women on the oxytocin gel (and without any estrogen) had completely normalized vaginal epithelium, which now looked like that of a younger healthy woman. None of the women on placebo had any benefit.

The scientists were dumbfounded. They thought maybe the estrogen levels would be high, but blood samples showed they weren't. Oxytocin does not boost estrogen or work through its receptors.

This is pretty amazing. This means oxytocin normalized, or "youthenized" if you will, vaginal epithelium like estrogen would, but without estrogenic action or without using estrogen or boosting estrogen levels in the blood. This translates into a huge, safe benefit for women who do not want to take any estrogen replacement, but want to improve their vaginal health, have less pain, more lubrication, and stay in intimacy sync with their mates.

This is very helpful to know. Go forth and educate your doctors.

Oxytocin protects breasts against cancer

Breasts make milk for a baby, so nature wants to protect breasts. When women orgasm, nature gifts the protection of the next generation, the milk source, the breasts. Rather a stunning circle when you see the whole biologic picture.

Dr. P. Cassoni and team from Department of Biomedical Sciences and Oncology, University of Turin, Italy, showed that oxytocin blocks many types of breast cancer cells from growing. Oxytocin boosts the good protective estrogen receptor that protects against breast cancer. And oxytocin boosts healthy immune function where most of our immune system is—in our gut wall. In other words, oxytocin acts like a *natural* Tamoxifen. This is pretty amazing. This means that it may be an adjunctive tool for women with a history of breast cancer to add to their other tools to prevent recurrence.

In *Hormone Deception,* I wrote about Dr. Timothy Murrell, a Professor from the University of Adelaide, who reported that oxytocin from orgasm flushes the breast of dangerous molecules that can cause cancer (free radicals, toxins, etc.). Dr. Murrel published studies showing that implants of oxytocin in rodent breast tissue caused regression of aggressive breast tumors.

139

Why oxytocin replacement?

If oxytocin is helpful for so many tissues, why wouldn't nature make sure we have enough of our own reserves of it? Why would we need replacement? That's a common question I hear from patients about oxytocin as well as many other hormones considered for replacement.

Remember, the ground rules have changed. Our air, food, and water daily bombard us with chemicals: plastics, pesticides, fertilizers, cosmetics, heavy metals that float onto our flower beds from far off China or India carried on mini whirlwinds that stay up in the air for over 30 years, remnants of chemicals long banned, and more.

These chemical hormones get into our bloodstream and hijack our natural hormones. Replacing hormones, when appropriate, elbows these hijackers out the receptors and reboots our own hormone signals. As well as our intimacy and bonding capabilities.

When we breathe in air with hidden chemicals, eat foods grown in soil with hidden contaminants, chomp on cheese that came in a shrink-wrapped package, and even wear cosmetics with hidden dyes and metals, we can get unintended exposure to these "enemies" of oxytocin. Our polluted planet contains some kryptonite-like chemicals that are assaulting our bonding and intimacy.

We have learned that hormones deliver signals to receptors. These receptors can get "clogged" with chemicals that literally block the hormone from performing its signaling service. These chemicals can block testosterone, progesterone, and estrogen, as well as thyroid, insulin, and adrenal signaling. Hormones are a family symphony. They act together. But only one hormone being blocked affects signaling in all the other hormones. Even if blood or saliva or urine test levels appear normal.

It is the same with oxytocin. I wondered how come so many of my patients responded so well to oxytocin replacement. When I surfed the literature, I learned that oxytocin receptors also can get inhibited by endocrine-disrupting chemicals. Remnants of PCBs, DDT, and other similar molecules can block the normal production, secretion, and signaling of oxytocin. There is even some discussion that synthetic oxytocin given during the birthing process might disrupt oxytocin receptors.

We have been thinking that our epidemic proportions of depression, anxiety, insomnia, and issues like inflammatory bowel disease were mainly due to our 24/7 stressful, under exercised, and junk food fed society. But apparently many of us are oxytocin insufficient, which may be contributing to our anxiety, gut woes, and, of course, to the detriment of our intimacy, mental health, and social and empathy skills.

How to fix this? Either through oxytocin replacement or through more cuddling, sex, and orgasm! Or both.

Aging also can impair receptor function. But if we become low in thyroid function as we age, we can get a script from our family doctor. Well, it's the same with oxytocin. Just as you can take prescribed thyroid replacement to feel healthier and have a better functioning thyroid, you can do the same with oxytocin. Some people need to take oxytocin replacement to feel better, to feel calmer, less stressed, more hopeful, but especially to feel more connected. And to have a better experience when connecting, especially in the bedroom. Oxytocin, among its many helpful aspects, is especially good at increasing the font size of orgasms.

Better living through chemistry.

Oxytocin testing and dosages

Meridian Valley Laboratory has a 24-hr urine assay for oxytocin, which is the only commercial test of its kind available in the U.S. at the time of writing this book. But oxytocin is so safe that you can try replacing it without testing. It can be prescribed by your doc and produced by a compounding pharmacy. Or you can buy over-the-counter (OTC).

Here are some typical dosages:

- Oxytocin is typically not dosed in mg. Instead it is dosed in units. IU/mg can change from one lot of oxytocin to the next.

- Dosage is everything. You may need to play around with the dose to get the optimal response.

- Delivery matters. Some people have been given oxytocin as oral lozenges. Most of the research uses nasal spray, which delivers oxytocin directly to the brain and seems to be more powerful.

- Typical dosages are: 10-30 IU in one or both nostrils once or twice a day

- Keep in fridge. Shake well before using as spray.

- To boost intimacy and orgasm: 30 minutes prior to intercourse, spray 24 IU in each nostril, and if necessary, repeat during intercourse.

- The vaginal gel dosing is in ranges from 80-120 IU per application.

- One pharmacy used dosing of 1gm QHS X 7 days, then twice a week thereafter with positive estrogen like results without any estrogen.

- I did notice over the last six years of using oxytocin replacement in patients (and myself), that some folks were amazingly improved, others weren't. Some got better for a while and then the benefits ceased. So I started to hang out in compounding pharmacies to learn how they do things.

Due diligence unveiled that the FDA allows a 10% +/− potency no matter what the label says. I discovered that just as there are various "grades" of food, like Whole Foods has very high-grade food and thus these items often have better taste but higher cost, so do hormones have different grades. Some companies can sell hormone products cheaper because their potencies are lower. Even though this isn't clearly reflected on the label.

When I worked once a week for almost six years at an integrative medical center in Tulsa, OK, I watched the pharmacists at CareFirst pharmacy in Broken Arrow, Oklahoma, work intelligently, professionally, and kindly with many hundreds of patients. I had repeatedly noticed that patients who used products from diverse sources got less consistent responses than when they obtained oxytocin from expert professional sources. This being the case, CareFirst and I teamed up to create a high-quality, over-the-counter (no prescription required), FDA compliant oxytocin product called OxySpray. We wanted to make sure a highly potent product was available for people to give oxytocin replacement an appropriate therapeutic trail. CareFirst ships to most states. Call 918-629-4474.

Oxytocin has been a personal game changer for me. I feel it is yet another tool to ward off possible recurrence of the breast cancer that I had over 20 years ago. It safeguards my gut wall and helps fight intestinal inflammation, helps ward off the diverticular diseases I had years ago. But most of all it has helped make my foundational perception of the world so much more even keel and positive!

I tell my patients oxytocin is "meditation up your nose."

What matters most is knowing that it may take some trial and error to see what dose and timing works best for you!

Warning: Oxytocin should NOT be used by infants or by pregnant or lactating moms, but it can be used in kids under the direct supervision of their pediatrician. There is a lot of research on the benefits of oxytocin for autism and social connectivity in children.

Studies show that giving oxytocin during labor (usually in a hospital setting) can negatively affect breastfeeding and possibly even create issues in the infant. So do not use oxytocin replacement during pregnancy or during labor without your gynecologist giving it to you, and do not use it during breastfeeding without the supervision of a medical expert.

During pregnancy, oxytocin use can cause abortion as it triggers labor. Although oxytocin is an essential hormone of lactation, use of it from a source outside of the mom has not been shown to help women having issues with lactation success or in the treatment of breast engorgement.

I would recommend you work with a physician about getting and taking oxytocin, but at this time, very few physicians know about the clinical applications or nuances of oxytocin replacement in any other setting but during birth. However, now you know.

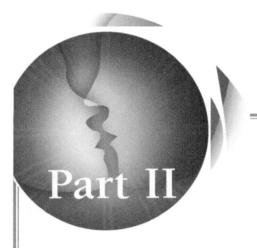

Part II

How To Do It
So Your Brain
and Partner
Love It

CHAPTER 9

Mid-Life Sex Mess Upgrades

I was sitting at Chuy's in Austin, Texas, an iconic restaurant, munching on my red cabbage, avocado, and hatch chili, when I heard a man complaining about losing all three of his ex-wives to menopause. That got my attention.

As each wife approached menopause, their sex life went south. All three women became angry, moody, and divorce material.

I gently approached him and explained I was a hormone expert. To his credit, Jim listened. I explained that when women age, their hormones tank and so does desire. But that desire, mood, and even relationships can be treated and rebooted by sensible hormone balancing and nutrition.

Jim took my card and was good on his word. The next time he got engaged, one of his presents was a joint session for both of them. It turns out you can teach an old dog new tricks.

We are learning how great sex protects our brain and overall health. But as many women enter mid-life, their enjoyment and ability to achieve fabulous sex can fly out the window.

This is scary.

- *She* wonders if she will ever enjoy sex or want it again.

- *He* wonders if she will ever enjoy sex or want it again.

- She may be married and worried about her relationship.

- She may be single and wonder if she missed her window.

She may start to have more anxiety, depression, and aches and pain and take medications for these, which make her want sex even less and make it almost impossible to achieve orgasm.

Yet balancing hormones, diet, lifestyle, and being able to want and share sex itself may help her feel less anxious and less depressed, hurt less, and not need drugs. And keep her bedroom jamming! There is HOPE.

Sex in sage ladies

Women can have sex issues in mid-life from perimenopause onward. Perimenopause is a *transition* time between when women can have babies and when they can't. It can last anywhere from one to ten years. During this time hormones start to roller coaster up and down. Women can feel and act in this up-and-down manner, too. Especially in the bedroom.

Women may experience bleeding changes (bleed more, spot, clot), and their vaginal tissues become drier, more sensitive, and more painful. Sex can start to hurt. It's hard to have fun if you hurt.

A woman can become emotional, anxious, or depressed. She can start to suffer with aches and pains and resistant (hard to shed) weight gain. Hurting more and feeling out of shape can lead to not wanting to be touched. Women start to release eggs less regularly each month so less progesterone is produced (it is produced mainly when the egg is released). This makes women have hot flashes, insomnia, and less sexual desire.

Earlier middle-age. On the whole, American women are going through perimenopause anywhere from two to fifteen years earlier than has occurred historically. Mid-life used to mean our 40s and 50s, though it can now mean even the 30s and sometimes the late 20s! (This data was presented to a San Diego OBGYN symposium in 2012.)

. . .

Chemicals outside of us can be messing with the hormones inside of us.

. . .

There are many reasons for this. A significant one is the environment. Many chemicals in the environment—in our air, food, and water—have potential endocrine-disrupting actions. Chemicals *outside* of us can be messing with the hormones *inside* of us. Earlier perimenopause puts women at an increased risk of mental issues and overall health issues and especially messes with sex life.

Often women are not correctly diagnosed when this is happening to them. But it may still be damaging both your sex lives, just when your starting-to-age brains would most benefit from sex hormone stimulation. When hormone blood levels are low enough that a woman has not menstruated for a solid year, she is officially *menopausal.*

Symptoms can get worse or calm down. A woman might have a new relationship with temperature as her body generates more heat. She suffers with hot flashes, during the night, the day, or both. Some women experience cold flashes immediately after the hot flashes. These flashes usually stop after a while, but some women can have these issues for up to a decade if not permanently.

In menopause, vaginal tissue gets thinner and less juicy, and sex can hurt and even cause bleeding.

These typical side effects of low hormones and aging can be all *reversed* with hormone replacement. But it's all in the dosage. When a woman gets a prescription for hormone therapy but still complains that the pleasure came back but not as much as before, she is not on the right dosage or adequate supportive nutrients, or she isn't digesting her nutrients optimally that help hormones work.

If you are a high risk patient (meaning you had breast or ovarian or uterine cancer or come from a family where many of the women had these issues) and are fearful of estrogen, you can try oxytocin gel. A vaginal gel made with oxytocin gives the same benefits to vaginal tissue as estrogen cream would, but without sending signals to estrogen receptors. So it's active similar to estrogens but without any estrogen signaling. So it's safe for high risk women.

Hysterectomies

Total hysterectomies (removal the uterus and both ovaries) put women into immediate menopause, putting them at increased risk for hormonal imbalances and deficiencies and, consequently, poor sex lives. But even removing only one ovary can make a woman's hormones come unglued. Sometimes even abdominal surgery, without removing the ovaries, can make a woman produce less hormones from then on. This is well documented in the literature but not appreciated by many doctors. And certainly not reported to many women. When these women see me and get on bioidentical hormone and nutritional treatment, their symptoms, overall health, and sex life are often improved within weeks.

In the year 2000, one out of every three American women by the age of 60 had had a hysterectomy. That is the same rate of adults, who are born after the year 2000, who now get diabetes. We call that a diabetes epidemic. Why don't we call the 400,000 hysterectomy surgeries performed a year, a hysterectomy epidemic? Hysterectomies are one of the most common surgeries performed in the U.S. There are a bit fewer hysterectomies performed today than in past decades, but still in large numbers that continue to threaten healthy hormone levels and intimacy capabilities.

Surgery scam. A study from my alma mater, the University of Michigan, published in the *Journal of Obstetrics and Gynecology* in January 2015, demonstrated that one out of every five women who got a hysterectomy didn't need it. This means she could have saved her uterus and hormones and sex life by more conservative means, which weren't suggested. Their research looked at the pathology reports of tissues removed and showed that two out of five women under the age of 30 who got hysterectomies did not actually have the issues for which they were diagnosed and recommended to get the hysterectomy.

This work has been replicated. That is the hallmark of science. Can what a study is saying been proven again and again by other research groups? An article in the *American Journal of Obstetrics & Gynecology* in 2015 found that many women who get hysterectomies were not offered alternative treatments first, and too often the pathology that was the supposed cause for the surgery was not found at time of the surgery. A study in *Obstetrics & Gynecology* in May 2016 found that ONLY 25% of women who got hysterectomies to stop their severe belly pain from endometriosis were actually found to have endometriosis when the surgeons went "in there."

Surgery robs T levels. Researchers from the Department of Gynecology and Obstetrics at Faculty Health Science in South Africa reported that the high rate of bilateral oophorectomy (removal of both ovaries) during hysterectomy markedly reduces circulating testosterone in both pre- and post-menopausal women. But they also showed that losing one ovary reduces testosterone blood levels, too. Sometimes a hysterectomy that doesn't remove an ovary but just the physician's act of touching and examining the ovaries makes them no longer produce adequate levels of testosterone.

Less testosterone means less sex drive, less bright brains, and often more aches and pains as well as anxiety. And commonly the pain and anti-anxiety meds used to treat these issues lower blood testosterone levels even more.

Mood and depression

The six most common symptoms of perimenopause and menopause are anxiety, depression, insomnia, resistant weight gain, more aches and pains, and *loss of libido and sexual satisfaction*. With hormone replacement prescribed individually and clinically "right on," many of these issues go away. Mood, sex, and weight often improve rapidly (within days to weeks). Then, when she wants and can enjoy sex more regularly, this helps sustain her hormone levels even more.

An aging female brain can be a moody thing. In fact, in the medical model, peri- and post-menopausal depressions are increasingly seen as new diagnosable subtypes of depression. Some literature even says that these may be life-long changes with no answers! Many of the medications used to treat anxiety and depression actually cause or worsen sexual dysfunction. They make it almost impossible to orgasm! Though if a woman needs to be on antidepressants, giving oxytocin along with it usually stops the sexual dysfunction issue.

But remember, fortification with strategic hormone replacement and healthier lifestyle habits, along with awakened sex, usually come rapidly to the rescue!

Bioidentical Hormone Therapy

Bioidentical hormone replacement (BHRT) often gets rid of severe anxiety, depression, and pain. It's certainly worth a clinical trail rather than going to meds first, which are demonstrated to have more dangerous side effects and often act to lower testosterone levels even more.

The literature clearly says that current medical treatments for peri- and post-menopausal *depression* have high failure rates. In other words, they don't work. Or they work for a while and then the women rebound fiercely when trying to go off them. That is because these treatments are not addressing the underlying root cause of the issues, which is usually hormonal, nutritional, and lifestyle imbalance.

In comparison to pharmaceuticals, individualized bioidentical hormone replacement often stops *all* these issues. With balanced BHRT, the woman can be back to her happier, friskier self within days to six weeks. And underneath, her heart, vocal chords, colon, bones, etc. are also benefitting.

Dr. K. Stephenson from the Women's Wellness Center in Tyler, Texas, reported that women treated with bioidentical hormones experienced less depression and could avoid antidepressant medication, compared to women not taking HRT. And they continued to enjoy sex, have better relationships, and reported less stress even though they all complained they had highly stressful lives.

Dr. Stephenson tested 75 peri- and post-menopausal women for estrogen, progesterone, and male hormone blood levels. Women who were deficient were treated with hormone replacement and then followed for three years. Most of the women did not need meds for sleep, high blood pressure, high cholesterol, high blood sugar, or anti-anxiety meds or therapy for libido loss. Why? Their balanced hormones kept them sane and purring. Markers of inflammation and heart health showed statistical improvement. Follow-up blood studies demonstrated statistical safety of the bioidentical hormones on the general health of these women.

Dr. Stephenson concluded that the negative effects reported about HRT were spin-offs from the Heart and Estrogen/Progestin Replacement Study I and the Women's Health Initiative studies. This makes sense as these studies used estrogen from horse's urine and synthetic progestins, not bioidentical estrogen and progesterone.

Safety of hormone replacement

In *Safe Hormones, Smart Women,* I explain the robust science behind the safety, sanity, and need for bioidentical hormone replacement. But there is an elegantly detailed article by a colleague of mine, Kent Holtorf MD, who in *Postgraduate Medicine* in 2009 faced this debate head on. Dr. Holtorf took a close look at the mass of scientific literature. He did a huge review from every scientific angle of published studies

(PubMed/MEDLINE, Google Scholar, and Cochrane databases) comparing the effects of bioidentical to synthetic hormones. And he then looked at the outcomes.

The articles showed that more women feel better when on bioidentical hormone replacement compared to synthetic versions. Women report feeling better and having more life satisfaction when hormone replacement contains bioidentical progesterone compared with therapies that contain a synthetic progestin.

Bioidentical hormones have some distinctly different and potentially opposite physiological effects compared with their synthetic counterparts (patented drugs that drug companies can own and profit from).

Holtorf clearly demonstrated:

- *Bioidentical progesterone* is associated with a *decreased* risk for breast cancer. In comparison, the use of *synthetic progestins* increases the risk. Synthetic progestins have a variety of negative effects on heart health, which are avoided with bioidentical progesterone.

- *Estriol* is unique compared to the other major estrogens (estradiol, estrone, and horse estrogen). Estriol carries less risk for breast cancer, although no randomized controlled trials have been documented. However, long-term human trials in Finland impressively show its safety. Estriol often reduces pain, reduces inflammation, and gives a sense of calm and balance to the body.

The data and clinical outcomes show that bioidentical hormones are associated with lower risks, including less risk of breast cancer and heart disease, and are more effective than their synthetic and animal-derived counterparts. (Go to http://drlindseyberkson.com/sexybrain/for P info)

Over-the-counter meds can assault your sexuality

In many women, the first two hormones to lower in perimenopause are testosterone and progesterone. Lower levels of these hormones

154

adversely affect mood, sex, and sleep on the most obvious levels, and brain, heart, and multi-tissue health on subtle tissue levels. Also, chemicals in today's environment are reducing testosterone and progesterone activity as many of them act to block their receptors. They are thus named antiprogestins and antiandrogens as they can block these critical hormone receptors.

A study of women showed that taking over-the-counter anti-inflammatory medications (NSAIDs like Ibuprofen), at the dose on the label, blocked progesterone activity enough to block fertility. But in the mid-life woman, this is enough to block sexual desire, sleep, and even brain function.

Pain as we age

Many of us, as well as doctors, regard pain as inevitable as we age. Many physicians, especially young ones who have not gone through seasonal life changes themselves, tell women they should just learn to live with their issues since they aren't getting any younger, or that they should just eat better and exercise more. Or take antidepressants and/or pain meds and learn to suck it up and age gracefully. But, I encourage my patients to never take *old* or *ill* for an answer.

In the olden days the aches and pains linked to aging were called *rheumatism*. Often, these types of pain are gone within days of balanced, sensible hormone therapy. This is because many aches and pains are actually due to insufficient levels of hormones, which are the major cause of aging. In fact, in a clinic I worked at where hormone therapy was mostly given through injections, many pains went away by the time the patient pulled into their driveway at home.

The authors of one article say hormone replacement should be a first line consideration to treat pain, before pain meds. And that many pain meds further lower hormone levels, making a downward spiral of suffering.

Many patients with severe and chronic pain don't get well with standard pain meds, including low to moderate dosages of opioids. These patients may have so much pain they are disabled, bedridden, or housebound. In this study, they looked at 61 patients with severe chronic pain and measured their hormone levels. Forty-nine patients demonstrated more than one hormone abnormality and seven patients showed a severe brain-hormone crosstalk abnormality.

The authors say that patients with chronic pain should all have their hormones tested. Deficient levels indicate that hormone replacement may be a helpful and a safe form of pain relief for these patients! And hormone therapy boosts sex desire and capability, while pain meds often do the opposite.

Pain med irony. Pain meds can lower hormone levels and cause more pain! Dr. Maddalena and co-workers from Italy wrote that *chronic pain itself can lower hormone levels.* They explain that *sex hormones are critical factors in how we experience pain.* Especially testosterone helps reduce our experience of pain. In fact, one reason women are more prone to painful sensations after procedures than men is that they have lower testosterone levels.

Dr. Maddalena says then the situation gets worse. Pain medication therapy itself, such as opioids, lowers testosterone blood levels. Thus, the chronic administration of painkillers, like oxycodone and hydrocodone, can cause testosterone deficiencies and worsen the pain. And worsen our libido! And the lower levels of testosterone contribute to rebound which makes these drugs even more difficult to stop taking.

These authors took surveys to see which pain clinics actually test hormone levels to address this root cause and treatment of pain. Almost zip.

Hey, instead of popping a pain pill, enjoy a quickie!

Sex as Mother Nature's pain reliever

Penile-vaginal stimulation has been shown to have pain-relieving properties. More so than sex by clitoral stimulation. It's not due to being distracted from the pain but rather from the hormones acting as pain relievers (testosterone and oxytocin) as well as the endorphins produced by lovemaking. All these are natural pain relievers.

It's odd and sad how medicine has made both practitioners and patients more comfy with drugs and procedures than with natural treatments, like hormone replacement. Dr. M. J. Brennan from The Pain Center of Fairfield in Connecticut, wrote that taking heavy pain meds for a long time is linked to pretty bad outcomes, such as potential peripheral edema, immune suppression, worsened pain, sleep apnea, and changes in endocrine function called *opioid endocrinopathy*, which can greatly reduce sexual function, decrease libido, cause infertility and issues with mood disorders, osteoporosis, and osteopenia.

Testing hormones and replacing those that are low can often reduce pain, while at the same time improving, not worsening, all the above-mentioned potential issues that pain meds can cause.

What does Dr. Brennan recommend? *Stop the meds and try hormone supplementation.* How often will you hear that from your doctors?

Vaginal cream with estriol and some testosterone, in the individualized dose for you, stops pain, increases lubrication, and makes pleasure soar. Can't use estriol? Try oxytocin. Don't want to use any hormones inside Miss Puss? Try a gel capsule of vitamin A.

Don't be fearful. Be smart.

Checklist for hormone health

- **Get your whole hormone family tested.** All hormones are a *family* that *function* and *dysfunction* together. If one family member is dysfunctional, this can affect your function or response in other hormones, so it is a good idea to get a complete blood test for the hormone family. See page 243 for a list of hormones to test.

  You can see a doctor to get tested or order your own hormone tests at Directlabs.com (they often have great

discounts). But you will need a doctor in the know to inter-
pret the results and to put you on a protocol that is effective,
and then monitor you with testing to see how you respond
and how you feel, both of which are crucial.

- **Clean up your diet.** Eat more plant foods, healthier fats,
avoid fried foods, eat more raw foods, and emphasize flax
seeds (super food, especially for hormones as they actually
promote the bioavailability of progesterone and help protect
the growth signals of estrogen), other seeds, nuts, avocados,
olives, organic cold pressed oils, more fish and less red meat,
grass fed meats (if you eat meat), healthy eggs, organic as
much as possible, etc. In other words, watch what you put
into your mouth.

- **Exercise more.** Less can be more when you use bursts of
high interval exercise, requiring less time to get a great work-
out. Google "high interval training" to find the appropriate
type or work with a trainer for several sessions. You can
accomplish a lot in fifteen minutes. We often neglect workouts when we convince ourselves that it takes an hour to
really do it right and then that seems too long to pull off.
Regular is the watchword. And bursts of high intensity,
where you *push yourself*, offer deep benefits. Fifteen minutes
daily is better than an hour twice a week.

- **Do Kegel exercises** as better pubococcygeal muscles help
you have better orgasms. Without training these muscles
they tend to get soft as you age and your orgasms take a hit.
These are for both men and women.

- **Eat fewer carbs.** Avoid refined sugars and foods with a high
glycemic index. If you do have desserts and other sugary
foods, have them as a treat and not regularly. See my books
Retraining Your Tongue and *Digestive Freedom*. Healthy carbs
are good, like veggies, quinoa, gluten-free steel cut oats,
buckwheat, nuts and seeds.

- **Get an evaluation by a digestive nutritional expert.** You need to balance your good-to-bad bacteria in the four-to-six pound organ of living organisms called your *microbiome*. Your gut health has a huge impact on your hormonal health. *If your gut bugs are off, so are your hormones, no matter your blood levels!* Attend to your gut to have healthier, sexier hormones!

- **Practice positive thinking.** As you clean out junk food from your diet, clean out junk food from your thoughts. Thoughts direct your moods. So do hormones, and the two together—intention for more positive thoughts along with BHRT—is a winner. Examples are: "I am safe, grateful, and healthy."

A really effective idea is to keep a gratitude journal and write down several things at the end of the day that you are grateful for. It doesn't have to be something that happened. Sometimes, especially if you're really down, being grateful for having a roof over your head, running water, or healthful food in your fridge can help reframe your thinking.

Way past menopause

I was in Houston one day and saw a poster on a wall advertising that it was the last day of a film festival in the museum district. I didn't even look at which movie was playing, but headed that way. I got there before anyone else and sat in the middle of the empty, upscale theater. Seniors with walkers, oxygen masks, and canes slowly drifted in. Turned out the movie was about being single in your eighties!

An elderly woman sat next to me, and we began to chat. She was 88 years old. She explained that when her third husband died, she found herself living alone in Mexico. She had battled five different cases of cancers and beat them all, and then moved on her own to Houston to be next to the best cancer institution in the world (MD Anderson). If she ever got cancer again, she intended to beat it again.

I asked her what she thought her secret was to staying so youthful.

She smiled and said, "All a woman needs are three things: your own money in the bank, a prescription for hormones on your shelf, and a vibrator in your drawer."

May the hormonal force be with you!

CHAPTER 10

Sex Needs Nutrients, Too

*J*eff was 32 and shy because no matter how pretty he thought a girl was, he couldn't perform. His doctor tested his hormone levels and they were fine. He saw a psychologist who helped him work through his family of origin issues, but he still couldn't perform. Jeff came in to see me at my office. Turns out that no one had ever asked him about his diet.

Jeff was a big fan of Mountain Dew soda. He consumed an entire case daily, along with seven or eight candy bars each day! All these chemicals and sugars were clogging his testosterone receptors and blocking the healthy cross talk between his gut bugs and testosterone signals. His lifestyle was ruining his hormone health, but no one had ever asked what he ate or drank. He cleaned up his diet, motivated by the thought of having a girlfriend. We did a receptor detox, a gut-boosting protocol, and gave him nutrients that helped boost testosterone health, especially zinc. In one month he felt amazing and within three months he had a girlfriend.

Sometimes it's lifestyle that's causing woes in the bedroom.

Radha was a yoga teacher who had been to all the hormone clinics in town and tried numerous protocols, and still had insomnia, hot flashes, and a poor *sex life. We ultimately found that her vegetarian diet was excessively high in grains that were blocking her ability to absorb minerals, like the mineral zinc, which is critical for healthy hormone signals. We gave her digestive enzymes, zinc supplementation, along with herbs to boost zinc absorption, and within two weeks she was as good as she had been several decades ago.*

In this chapter you will learn that our intimacy, our ability to have and share love, is being assaulted from our outside toxic environment and our inside (gut) toxic environment. In this chapter, a number of my past books (on digestion, the environment and hormones) converge in your boudoir.

Hormones depend on nutrients

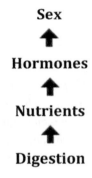

Sex

Hormones

Nutrients

Digestion

Hormones and *intimacy* all lean on *nutrition*.

- *Sex* and *hormones* depend on nutrients.

- *Nutrients* depend on *digestion*.

- This new field is called *nutritional endocrinology*. It is the understanding that your hormones, nutrients, food, and gut health all interact and affect each other. And your sex and love life.

By nutrition, I mean food and nutrients. By digestion, I mean the health of your digestive support team (stomach acid, digestive enzymes, gut flora, and gut wall).

Remember, receptors are shaped like a satellite dish. Their molecular appearance looks somewhat like a deep bowl. Hormones swim into this. But this bowl-shaped receptor has to be filled with nutrients for the hormonal emailing to work "just right." Hormones can't do what they are designed to do without adequate nutrition.

Local tissue levels of critical nutrients go hand in hand with healthy hormonal functioning. The receptor bowl needs to be flush with zinc, magnesium, B vitamins, and even amino acids. When these are present in optimal amounts, signaling takes place just right. If these nutrients are insufficient, if digestion is not so hot, then hormone signals can be hit or miss. And you just don't feel like it, or enjoy it.

These local nutrients help the receptor receive the critical messages from hormones and translate them to your genes. They help the messages be pulled into the receptor. They help the messages be translated. And they oversee the duration of how long the signals are sent.

Too many or too few nutrients and your hormonal timing and signaling can go kaflooey.

Nutrients are part of where the hormonal rubber meets the hormonal road. They allow hormone messages to be received, read, and delivered.

Most doctors don't know this and don't take nutrition into account when prescribing or figuring out hormonal issues and responses to treatment.

Sometimes natural or even prescribed hormones don't help sexual woes because people are deficient in nutrients inside the receptors, or these people may have digestive issues that don't allow for the nutrients to be optimally absorbed into the cells that live inside the receptors.

Any cogent approach to hormones and sex means that you have gone through a checklist of associated factors that might be contributing to your sexual woes. Fixing these may be part of your sexual success story.

Zinc

Not enough zinc? Your feet may stink. That's an old adage of one of the many symptoms of zinc deficiency. But one of the biggest deficiency signs of zinc is when hormones are not working right. Without adequate zinc, you can have enough blood levels of sex hormones, but they might not get *grabbed* into the receptor to deliver email.

Estrogen, testosterone, and progesterone must have adequate zinc to deliver their signals.

Zinc is also directly related to reproductive potential. Low levels of zinc increase the risk of infertility in men, while zinc supplementation improves fertility.

Zinc is found in whole, natural foods, which many people don't eat. Often, as people age, they can become deficient in stomach acid, which is necessary to help digest zinc. Pollutants in air, food, and water can hamper our ability to use zinc. Endocrine disruptors can damage the zinc fingers that *pull* sex hormone messages into genes.

．　．　．

Heavy metals in the environment (from cigarette smoke to dust to other types of contamination) can sabotage zinc fingers.

．　．　．

Heavy metals in the environment (from cigarette smoke to dust to other types of contamination) can sabotage zinc fingers by bumping zinc out of the way and inserting cadmium or lead. This then blocks hormone signals. You might be inadvertently exposed to third-hand smoking. This is smoke exposure that you did not inhale, but has settled on hair, clothing, pillowcases and other surfaces, that you later inhale. Third-hand smoke can still ding your hormonal and sexual prowess.

Part of the process of digesting and using nutrients and responding to hormones is called *methylation*. This process can also be hampered by endocrine-disrupting pollutants.

I was a reader for a consensus statement on the causes of the type 2 diabetes epidemic by the World Health Organization. One of the many new causes of type 2 diabetes discussed in this paper is pollution. Cadmium, potentially in air, food, or water, gets into our bodies and displaces zinc. Insulin receptors then become disabled because the zinc finger gets thwarted, and insulin has trouble delivering its email.

Remember, all hormones are a family. If one family member is not working, it can disrupt the whole family. If your insulin is not working right, it may disrupt your sex hormones, like testosterone or estrogen. Even if your blood work appears healthy.

It's easy to become zinc deficient, or zinc malfunctioning, which puts the kibosh on hormone health. The end result is that you miss out on great sensations, sizzle, and sex.

I believe that environmental disruption of zinc fingers is one growing cause of the increase of hormonal disorders occurring at younger ages and the reason that so many are experiencing sexual problems (other than obesity, insulin resistance, and type-2 diabetes).

Earlier hormonal issues on the rise including environmental castration

At the clinic where I work in Cedar Park, Texas, we are seeing an epidemic of hormonal issues in teenage girls (polycystic ovarian syndrome) as well as earlier and messier (more symptoms and issues) perimenopause in middle-aged women.

At a symposium in San Diego in 2012, we learned that American women are going through perimenopause anywhere from two to fifteen years earlier than women before us. Practitioners are seeing more sexual dysfunction at earlier ages across the board. A National Institute of Health urologist (at a functional medicine meeting I helped teach in Las Vegas in February 2015) said low levels and malfunctioning of testosterone are being reported in men in their twenties. It's a real epidemic. Part of the reason may be all the factors (pollutants, antibiotics, gut woes, poor diet, lack of digestive enzymes and/or stomach acid, age, and on and on) that are making the zinc fingers unable to assist in the delivery of the critical hormonal email.

Anyone with sexual issues needs to be evaluated for zinc. Zinc should be assessed at the *intracellular* level (zinc levels *inside* cells), as well as doing a digestive evaluation, because zinc depends heavily on optimal digestion to be reduced to a proper electronic state to enter the cells. If you have gut issues, you may not absorb enough zinc to keep your hormones humming.

Vitamin B6: our hormone signaling metronome

Other local nutrients are needed for healthy hormone signaling, such as iodine, magnesium, protein, and especially vitamin B6.

Vitamin B6 is like a metronome for sex steroid signaling, especially estrogen and testosterone. It controls how long the hormones deliver their signal. It also has input into the metabolism and balance of these hormones. Vitamin B6 also helps optimize signaling of cortisol (which directs the crucial anti-inflammatory actions of the body), and it's looking like this is also true for the pro-hormone vitamin D.

Dr. Alan Gaby, a lifelong friend and colleague and a highly respected physician in nutritional medicine, wrote one of my favorite books, *The Doctor's Guide to Vitamin B6* (Rodale Press, 1984). Dr. Gaby shows us how environmental pollutants—found in our air, food, water, and pharmaceuticals—are putting vitamin B6 cellular levels under siege. Since vitamin B6 is the major orchestrator of healthy hormone *timing*, it becomes apparent how contemporary "environmental-isness," with its plethora of chemicals, is making it difficult for our hormones stay in rhythm.

In other words, vitamin B6 helps keep signaling at its optimal tempo. Environmental pollutants and junk-food diets can deplete vitamin B6 and create hormonal cacophony and, thus, sexual dysfunction.

Diet/hormone link

A man or woman with poor digestion or who is undernourished may be flush with hormones, but these hormones may not be able to deliver emails to the genes successfully. A poor diet, doing a bad job of digesting food, or issues with hidden food intolerances and leaky gut problems can all play an unappreciated role in hormonal and sexual dysfunction. A middle-aged man or woman may be deficient in stomach acid (by sixty years old, 70 percent of people are deficient in stomach acid) or other digestive enzymes (like bile or proteolytic enzymes) and not be able to completely digest critical nutrients in his or her diet.

Many practitioners do not consider nutrition, digestion, and exposure to chemicals as part of the hormonal mix.

This is unfortunate and promotes non-optimal health care when, clearly, hormones and sexual health depend on nutrients right down to the atomic and molecular levels. This is another reason it's accurate to refer to sex as a "nutrient," since it is part of the constellation of actions of so many of our other nutrients.

Hormone resistance (not just to *thyroid* and *insulin*, but also to our *sex hormones*)

It is now well documented that contemporary American women are entering perimenopause earlier than generations before. The consensus theory is that this is partly due to environmental pollutants that can clog sex steroid receptors.

Due to the flexible, wide-open shape of receptors, they are easily filled up with compounds that compete with hormones, such as environmental chemicals that enter from air, food, water, cosmetics, pharmaceuticals, and even from excess levels of other hormones. In this way, hormone receptors can get clogged and can't receive hormone signals. *Clogged receptors* and *insufficient levels of supportive nutrients* play a role in hormones not being able to deliver their signals. This is called *hormone resistance*.

Hormonal resistance can happen with any hormone, not just the two most commonly recognized cases of resistance, which are insulin and thyroid resistance. There can be *testosterone resistance* and even *progesterone resistance*, which can play a role in a lack of hormone health and ultimately lead to decreased desire and enjoyment of sex. Not to mention a higher risk for brain fog and dementia.

There is an increased incidence today of undiagnosed and unrecognized hormonal resistance due to the plethora of endocrine-disrupting compounds in our world. I wrote about this in my book *Hormone Deception: How Our Environment Is Hijacking and Deceiving Our Hormones and What to Do About It.*

- Great sex requires healthy sex hormone receptors.

- Receptors need to be available.

Just like both persons in a relationship need to be emotionally available, receptors need to be ready and open for business to accept hormonal signals, not already occupied by competing pollutants, plastics, pesticides, heavy metals and more. So a responsive receptor is a healthy available receptor. Great receptor function requires a healthy gut, a healthy diet, and receptor function.

The vitamins most required are B vitamins. Too much sugar, a bad diet in general, environmental pollution, and many dyes found even in medications, repetitive rounds of antibiotics, can rob your body of B vitamins, especially if you don't refortify yourself daily. The ability to methylate requires natural folate, not folic acid, which is the synthetic version of folate and has its own issues (vitamin B12 and SAMe help with this) along with minerals like iodine and magnesium.

Receptor Detox

In-the-scientific-know physicians, like Dr. Jonathan Wright (often called the Father of Bioidentical Hormones) and myself, often put patients on receptor detoxification programs prior to hormone replacement programs or if they are not responding to the hormone replacement they have already been taking in order to give them a better chance to benefit from the hormones. This is a protocol designed to clean out receptors too filled with potentially competing substances (scientifically called *competitive inhibitors*) to accept hormonal email appropriately.

. . .

Cleaner Receptors = Healthier Hormones = Deeper
Intimacy = More Brain Power

. . .

The scientific ability to detox and to prove that chemicals can be removed from fat cells, membranes, and receptors came from original research on firemen who were exposed to chemicals on the job and became ill. Specific protocols were developed to clean these chemicals out of their bodies and this detox was shown to be effective in getting those gallant guys feeling better and back on the job once again.

Receptor detox is based on:

1. *Improving cell membrane fluidity,* especially in mitochondria.

2. *Boosting the P450 enzyme system helps "rinse" pollutants* out of the local membranes, the liver, and eventually our of the body.

3. *Rebooting local gut and microbiome health* helps continue the rinsing of pollutants out of the body and reinforces testosterone and estrogen signaling.

4. *Supplying the nutrients, protein, and specific foods* that help improve lymph flow and receptor dynamics to help hormones do their magic exactly right.

5. *Removing stressor foods that sabotage* hormone health and signaling.

Berkson's 10-Day Receptor Detox

This is a program to help remove pollutants that can harm hormonal health, including desire and your capacity for intimacy, as well as improve your brain's responsiveness to cognition-boosting hormones.

When to do it?

- *Yearly.* Several times a year to boost intimacy enjoyment and skills. Detoxing several times a year is optimal as we are exposed to endocrine-disrupting chemicals in our air, food, and water 24/7.

- *Before conception.* This detox can safely be done before conception to protect pregnancy hormones and the health of the future baby. It is too strong to be used during pregnancy. A gentler and more personalized pregnancy detox can be done while pregnant, but must be professionally and closely monitored.

- *HRT.* Prior to any hormonal therapy replacement programs to make them safer and more effective.

- *Hormonally driven disorders.* When you have hormonal issues like PMS, PCOS, or menopause problems.

- *Resistant weight.* If you want to lose weight safely.

- *Optimize health.* To boost overall health.

- *Anti-aging.* Staying "cleaner" keeps you "younger."

Ideally you work with a professional to have this detox individualized and monitored. Watch the detox webinar here: http://drlindseyberkson.com/resources, then reach Dr. Berkson at dlberkson@gmail.com to set up a consult.

What you will need

Food: Whole flaxseeds, chia seeds, walnuts, wild fish, grass-fed lamb, turkey, chicken, blueberries, stevia, colorful veggies like red cabbage, broccoli sprouts, white onions, yellow onions, red grapes, kale, curly parsley, limes, green beans, spinach, mung bean sprouts, beets, beet greens, daikon radish, red radish, green scallions, olive oil in glass bottle, organic whole coffee beans, organic pomegranate concentrate (for your Sweep Drink), seeds, nuts.

- Eat only *organic* as we are trying to remove pollutants out of your body. Taking in pollutants from non-organic food reduces the effectiveness of the detox program.

- No grains except quinoa or buckwheat groats or pasta in moderation.

- Onions are one of the most anti-inflammatory foods. If you are not reactive or allergic to onions, add them generously to your diet.

- Have *at least* 2 tablespoons of broccoli sprouts twice a day; they are a food probiotic.

- Have at least 5 to 9 servings of colorful veggies a day.

- *Hari hachi bu*: Leave the table when you are 75% full. Eat smaller portions than usual so your body has more energy to detox. Take 3 deep breaths before eating. Eat slowly and chew well. Practice mindful eating.

- No refined, processed, fried, barbequed or inorganic foods. Charred veggies are fine. No fast food. No restaurant food unless it is at an organic, healthy restaurant. You can do this more easily by avoiding foods in boxes and cans.

- While detoxing, no gluten or dairy (milk from an animal). If you use nut or grain milks, make sure they are *un*sweetened. Plain versions often still contain sweeteners.

- Sweeteners: No refined sugars, artificial sweeteners, or high fructose corn syrup. No honey and agave syrup. Stevia and xylitol are okay.

Supplements:

- *Bentonite liquid* – Sonnes #7 (purchase online)

- *Soluble fiber* (with nothing else added)

- *Evening primrose oil*, 2 capsules (500 mg) with breakfast

- *LivCo* (by Standard Process), 3 with breakfast and dinner. It is high in milk thistle and rosemary compounds that help the liver handle the chemicals that are released during the detox.

- *Ca/Mg butyrate* supplements, to be used with coffee enema

- *Watercress extract* pills or powder, 5 with each meal 3 times a day

- *Chlorella* supplements, 5 with each meal 3 times a day

- *Iodoral iodine* supplement, 12.5 mg take with one dinner (this helps the lymph move the hormone acting pollutant through your body). You cannot continue this high dose indefinitely. This is only for these 10 days.

- *DHA Ultra Nordic Natural*, 2 with dinner

- *Pure Encapsulation 650 mineral*, without copper or iron

- *Oxytocin nasal spray*, 20 to 30 IU of nasal spray of oxytocin in each nostril twice a day to heal leaky gut, prevents what is released from re-entering the body and reduces inflammation. On rising, get oxytocin from fridge, shake, and spray into each nostril. This helps to keep you feeling amazingly good! OTC oxytocin nasal spray (available from CareFirst Pharmacy, but not to all states). There is a less potent source that is still OTC, called *Oxyluv*, available on Amazon or you can get it by a script from your doctor. If you can't get this, use 1000 mg of *chanca piedra* twice a day with food.

Other: You can find an enema bag in the feminine section of Walgreens. Distilled water for coffee enemas. Skin brushes are available online.

Recipes

Potato Skins: Bake organic Russet potatoes, cool them, and remove much of the white potato inside; coat the outside with olive oil and broil, add granulated garlic and sea salt and cut into croutons or use the entire skin like a tortilla.

Parsley Limeade: Small handful of parsley, 1 tsp. of organic dried parsley flakes, juice of 4-6 limes, 3-4 Tbsp. of stevia to taste, 8-10 ice cubes and a glass of water and blend till you cannot see anymore parsley bits or hear ice cubes hit the side of the Vita Mix. Drink twice a day, with or without meals. It stays in fridge for two days but needs to be stirred before consuming.

Daily Morning Seed Cereal: Using a small inexpensive coffee grinder (you can purchase at most grocery stores), each morning grind and put in a bowl:

- 1 TB of flaxseeds
- 1 TB of 5 walnuts
- 1 TB of chia seeds
- 1 heaping TSP of hemp seeds
- Add vanilla milk alternative, like unsweetened vanilla almond, coconut, flax, or soy milk.
- Add stevia to taste.
- And a few berries (optional).

The lignins from flaxseed help clear the pollutants out.

Flaxseed is also the one food that boosts 2-methoxyestradiol, which helps keep hormones healthier and more in balance.

Clean Sweep Drink: 3 times daily in between meals:

Add each below to ½ glass of water, stir, drink right away, then follow with a whole glass of water (filtered water).

1. 1 TB Bentonite liquid Sonnes #7

2. 1 TB of soluble fiber

3. (Optional) 1 TB of sugar-free organic pomegranate concentrate

Dessert: You can choose to eat the breakfast seed cereal again after dinner as a dessert. Or place a dab of maple syrup on a walnut and enjoy. Another option is a bowl of blueberries with lemon zest, handful of walnuts, and stevia or a dash of maple syrup.

Activities

Meal frequency affects receptor health. You can promote better insulin receptor health by having longer times in between meals, along with less snacking and avoiding eating three hours prior to bed time. Insulin receptor health affects global receptor health. For best results, I recommend that you eat two meals a day without snacking in between for optimal receptor function. But not everyone feels good eating this infrequently. Thus, three daily meals are offered in case you cannot accomplish this, and to give you extra meal ideas. The concept of "three meals a day" and snacking has led to a more obese and hormonally unhealthy nation. Less food and more time between meals is the new goal of a healthy diet for longevity and hormonal brilliance.

Coffee enema (before dinner): Most people sleep better with a coffee enema. If you have a hard time sleeping, do the enema in the morning or whenever you can).

- Must be organic and freshly ground. Can be made ahead of time, lasts in fridge for 3 days. Cool down to room temperature. Empty one capsule of butyrate into 2 cups of coffee in enema bag.

- Place coffee inside you, lie on back with feet up on side of bathtub, retain in for 10 to 15 minutes or as long as comfy. If you have to release immediately, then repeat.

- Every other night increase the number of butyrate capsules emptied into the coffee, so by the 10th night there are 5 capsules in the coffee.

Skin brushing: Purchase a skin brush. Brush skin from your torso out towards your extremities; shower afterwards. Skin brush and shower twice a day. Your skin is an organ of detox and this helps promote detoxification.

Exercise: at least once a day in a way that causes you to sweat (for example 15 minutes on an exercise bicycle in which you have several 30 second bursts of high intensity going all out where your heart rate goes up and your metabolism speeds up. This helps move the chemicals out of your fat cells and clear them out of your body. If you cannot do this, then you most likely need to work with a professional to do a gentler detox.

Steam and Sauna: You can opt to sit in a steam room or sauna for regular sessions throughout the detox, which heightens the detox. Do not do this if you have any cardiac conditions or contraindications.

The Rainbow Diet

During the 10-day detox program, we add a different colored food each day to supply the benefits of that particular polyphenolic pigment. This gets you to eat a rainbow diet that further facilitates the detox. Plant pigments in veggies give various benefits to your body. So eating a rainbow diet means you try to consume as many colorful, diverse plant foods as you can. This is NOT mandatory if you can be good about eating many diverse veggies foods daily. This is to get you familiar with doing so. It's up to you.

On days 6 – 10, repeat the colors of days 1 – 5.

Desert ideas are optional, or enjoy them as snacks.

This is educational; to merely give your ideas and creativity of how to eat diverse and colorful plant foods.

- **Day 1**: *Blue, purple, indigo*—blueberries, eggplant, small purple potatoes, and at least ¼ c. of shredded purple cabbage.

- **Day 2**: *Orange and red*—beets, sundried tomato paste, carrots, yams, sweet potatoes, red radishes, strawberries, blackberries, goji berries, pimento, red peppers.

- **Day 3**: *White*—cauliflower, white onions, scallions, garlic, potato skins, white/green cabbage, daikon radish.

- **Day 4**: *Green*—have at least 3 leafy greens (kale, parsley, lettuce), and green beans, snap peas, mung bean sprouts

- **Day 5**: *Yellow*—make sure you get some yellow or red squash, some yellow peppers, some garlic, or some yellow onions.

After the 10-day detox:

Consume broccoli sprouts once a day

Do 3 more coffee enema every 3 days.

Slowly add back in other foods and notice how you feel. Awareness, and then acting on it, is the basis of wisdom, especially in how you learn to keep yourself vibrant and well.

Daily Charts

DAY 1: Blue, Purple, Indigo	Breakfast	Mid-morning	Lunch
	Casein-free whey powder with frozen blueberries and unsweetened flaxseed milk /morning cereal /coffee or tea optional	Sweep drink followed by parsley limeade	Turkey on top of avocado with kalamata olives or tapenade, purple potato skins or potato skin croutons, salad with grated coleslaw, onions, mayo, very slight xylitol, 2 TB broccoli sprouts
	Mid-afternoon	**Dinner**	**Before Bed**
	Sweep drink **Snack:** mixed raw nuts with dried blueberries (without sugar)	Black exotic rice, fish or chicken, sautéed beet greens, lime, granulated garlic, sea salt, veggies; purple grapes, parsley limeade, 2 TB broccoli sprouts **Dessert** – blue berries, lemon zest, stevia, a few chopped walnuts	Sweep drink/ coffee enema/ skin brushing

DAY 2: Orange, Red	Breakfast	Mid-morning	Lunch
	Parsley limeade/ morning cereal	Sweep Drink	Salmon salad with grated red pepper, red radishes, sundried tomato paste, diced sweet onions, celery, capers and mayo, 2 TB broccoli sprouts.
	Mid-afternoon	**Dinner**	**Before Bed**
	Sweep Drink **Snack** – mixed nuts with dried goji and cranberries	Buckwheat pasta & sautéed thinly slicked yam with sun dried tomato paste, Parsley limeade, 2 TB broccoli sprouts. Dessert: several slices of mandarin oranges & bananas dipped in raw hemp seeds & cocoa nibs	Sweep Drink/ Coffee enema

DAY 3: White	Breakfast	Mid-morning	Lunch
	Smoothie with casein free whey powder /morning cereal	Sweep Drink and Parsley limeade	Grass-fed lamb burger made with lots of diced veggies and white onions and olives, salad, 2 TB broccoli sprouts
	Mid-afternoon	**Dinner**	**Before Bed**
	Sweep Drink	Gluten-free pasta & veggies, Baked chicken or fish with olive tapenade on top, Parsley limeade, 2 TB broccoli sprouts	Sweep drink/ coffee enema

DAY 4: Green	Breakfast	Mid-morning	Lunch
	Parsley limeade/ morning cereal	Sweep drink	Chicken, salad with grated zucchini, diced parsley & kale, 2 TB of dried parsley, olive oil and sea salt, half an avocado with sprinkled cayenne pepper on top, 2 TB broccoli sprouts.
	Mid-afternoon	**Dinner**	**Before Bed**
	Sweep drink Snack: roasted wasabi soy nuts	Parsley limeade, tofu & veggies (green beans, beet greens, diced celery and diced sugar snap peas, parsley) limeade, 2 TB broccoli sprouts. Dessert: frozen green grapes with a dash of cashew paté (blended raw cashews, water, vanilla, stevia or xylitol)	Sweep drink/ coffee enema

DAY 5: Yellow	Breakfast	Mid-morning	Lunch
	Casein free whey powder with frozen kiwi & peaches & unsweetened non dairy milk/morning cereal	Sweep drink	Stuffed yellow peppers with Cashew pate (raw cashews blended with water, lemon, several TB of dehydrated onion flakes, sea salt, gluten free pasta) & a dash of umeboshi plum paste topped with 2 TB broccoli sprouts.
	Mid-afternoon	**Dinner**	**Before Bed**
	Sweep drink **Snack:** handful of olives.	Cod fish with smoked paprika, ginger, olive oil & gluten-free soy sauce, sautéed grated yellow squash, yellow onions, mung bean sprouts & gluten-free noodles in chicken broth & herbs, Parsley limeade, 2 TB broccoli sprouts. Dessert: slices of papaya with lime	Sweep drink/ coffee enema

Daily Supplements

With Breakfast	With Lunch	With Dinner	Before Bed
5 watercress; 5 chlorella; 2 Evening Primrose oil; 3 LivCo; 1 Orthodigest, 1 Pure Encapsulation 650 minerals, 1 Orthodigest Methyl Bs; oxytocin spray	5 watercress extract; 5 chlorella; 1 Orthodigest; 1 Pure Encapsulation 650 minerals	5 watercress, 5 chlorella, 1 Orthodigest, 1 Pure Encapsulation 650 minerals, 2 DHA Ultra Nordic Natural; 1 Iodoral; 3 LivCo; oxytocin spray	1 butyrate capsule in coffee; Increase every other day until doing 5 capsules by day 10.

Walnut Paté

Walnuts are a magical food. You should add 2 Tbsp. of paté daily to one of your meals or snack during the 10-day detox. Or simply snack on a handful of walnuts. I especially like them with a few organic purple grapes.

Walnuts contain ellagic acid. Ellagic acid promotes a healthy and diverse microbiome (good gut bugs) and healthy gut wall. Ellagic acid also tamps down the out-of-control growth of cancer cells.

Secondly, walnuts contain melatonin. Melatonin is a robust cancer fighter. When you eat walnuts, there has been proven to be an almost immediate increase of blood melatonin concentration.

When I worked as a hormone scholar at a hormone think tank at Tulane University, researchers there demonstrated that melatonin is secreted at night, not just to help us sleep, but also to help us tamp down cancer cells while we sleep. Melatonin has been shown to be effective against almost 60 cancer cell lines.

Walnuts also protect the brain. Walnuts protect the brain against the normal "hits" of aging produced by oxidative stress. Walnuts have also been shown to nullify the toxicity of metals and other contaminants linked to brain aging.

Walnut paté is a very bioavailable form of walnuts, as well as being delicious and fun to make and eat.

Walnut paté is great on Nancy's Gone Crackers, on veggies like celery and slices of red pepper, and even great as a side dish with salads, chicken, fish, or beans. It is also great placed inside Romaine lettuce leaves with a dash of umeboshi plum paste on top (promotes healthy microbiome) and some broccoli sprouts on top. Healthy to the max! Tasty to the maxed out!

Walnut Paté recipe:

Put in a Vita Mix:

- 1 stalk of celery (keep the leaves on)
- ½ to one carrot
- 1-½ cups of organic raw walnuts
- 1/3 sweet or yellow onion (onions are one of the best anti-inflammatory foods. I love onions so much I put in an additional TB of dehydrated onions.)
- 2 TB of gluten-free soy sauce
- 2 small cloves of garlic and/or 1 TSP of raw garlic granules
- juice of 1-2 limes
- sea salt to taste

1 heaping TSP of organic dried parsley flakes (especially high in the flavonoid apigenin, which helps to kill supposedly immortal cancer cells)

Olive oil. Add enough to blend to the consistency that tastes good to you.

More Options:

For more flavor zing:

- 1 TSP of smoked paprika

- 1/2 TSP of cayenne pepper.

- Adding turmeric is good in that it helps to reduce polyp growth.

- Often I add even more dehydrated onion flakes (I like a very onion-y flavor oh so much).

For a creamier consistency:

- *Non-dairy cheese addition*: Sometimes I add a chunk of the non-dairy cheese, Daiya wedge (only wedge, not purchased as grated or in slices as this cheese in these forms do not taste anywhere near as good). Adding this to the mix makes a chunky cheese-y very cool flavor and creamy texture.

- You can add a few Tbsp. of water. That makes it too creamy for me but some folks adore it.

CHAPTER 11

Prevent the Big "A" With the Big "O"

*S*uzanne was a student at the local college but her memory was shot. She was fearful she wouldn't be able to pass her courses and graduate. When I assessed her situation, she was so anxious about school that she and her boyfriend were only seeing each other two times a month and only making love once a month or sometimes once every two months.

I explained the brain-boosting benefits of regular sex with your regular guy. They thought I was a cool doc to give such a cool prescription and they agreed to try it. So they made a point to have three short and sweet date nights a week.

Within two months, with no other changes at all, Suzanne reported better memory, sharper focus, and more calm and courage. Doing "it" helps you make it in other arenas of your life.

·   ·   ·

Now that we are living longer, the biggest fear has become our brain health.

·   ·   ·

The number one fear for many people used to be of getting cancer. Now that we are living longer, the biggest fear has become our brain health. Will we get dementia or Alzheimer's? Will we be able to continue to think, focus, and remember? It turns out that hormone levels in the blood and the brain and stimulation that occurs during orgasm have a lot to do with maintaining healthy brain function and avoiding cognitive decline.

We have heard for years that if you masturbate too much (or at all), you will go blind, and, if you have too much sex you will meander about in a brain fog. As it turns out, nothing could be further from the truth.

Sex and your brain are a match made in heaven.

Should doctors recommend sex?

Sex supplies a banquet for the hippocampus—sperm, rich in estrogen, along with oxytocin and the testosterone jolt from cuddling and touching and entry.

A group of scientists at a center for psychological research in Coventry, England, wanted to see if doctors should be recommending frequent pleasure-filled sex to their patients to help ward off the dementia epidemic as the aging demographic surges (published in *Age Ageing* in January of 2016). They looked at almost 7,000 men and women, aged 50 to 90 years old, how often they had intercourse, and how well their brains functioned by testing abilities to remember and state numbers and words in various order. After adjusting for age, education, wealth, physical activity, depression, cohabiting, self-rated health, loneliness, and quality of life (in other words, nothing else was influencing the statistics), there were *significant* (beyond chance) associations between how often you do it and how you think.

Sexually active men and women had significantly better cognition. They had higher scores on the number sequencing and recall tests than sexually inactive men and women. In other words, the more these folks made love, the healthier their gray matter got.

Other studies agree. A large review of sex studies, conducted out of the Netherlands, found that most studies historically had been looking at the question: *once we lose our wits, do we keep having sex?* But three studies looked at healthy maturing folks to see how sex preserved their aging wits. The trend of the results showed that older people who continue to engage in sexual activity have overall better cognitive functioning, focus, memory and mood.

So, yes, doctors *should* talk about your sex life and consider prescribing sex for better brain cognition!

The hippocampus—the home of "me"

The hippocampus in the brain is the home of the three M's: *memory, motivation,* and *ME-ness.* It consolidates short- and long-term memory and spatial orientation (where am I and why and how did I get here, as in why did I walk into this room or where is my car in the parking lot?). It also is the repository for your sense of *self-awareness*—who you are and how you keep on being who you want to be, and how to accomplish everything you hope to do. I feel like the hippocampus is the physical analogy of the soul, the very epicenter of ourselves.

Nature prioritizes the hippocampus. We know this. Why? All cells need *mitochondria.* These are the energy furnaces inside all cells to provide energy for any function the cell has to do. But nature places the most mitochondria inside cells that require the most energy because they are the most critical for life. Hippocampal cells (in your tiny, mighty hippocampus) have the highest volume of mitochondria of any other cell in the entire human body. Nature wants to make sure that these clump of cells don't suffer any glitches for as long as possible.

The hippocampus is small; it's less than 1/200 the size of blood vessels. Yet the hippocampal levels of male and female hormones (testosterone and estrogen) are much higher than the levels found in the bloodstream. Why? The hippocampus *eats* T and E signals for food.

The hippocampus is lined with thousands of male and female hormone receptors to receive these critical hormone signals. The hippocampus is a veritable hotbed of Venus and Mars activity.

. . .

The hippocampus is a veritable hotbed of Venus and Mars activity.

. . .

Estrogen and testosterone encourage and promote nerve communication (neuroplasticity) and the ability of the hippocampus to do what it is supposed to do—remember and keep you "who" you are. The more appropriately robust your blood levels of testosterone and estrogen are, the more the hippocampus hums along. And then so do you.

All this is backed by science. But the science is new and not well known by many practitioners, even gynecologists, or urologists, or endocrinologists. Or sex therapists. Or psychologists, pastors, or rabbis.

The hippocampus ages

As teenagers, we are full of ourselves. When we are going through puberty, our bodies are awash in the highest amount of hormones we will ever have (except during pregnancy). We think we know more and better than everyone else, especially parents, because our hormones are creating a feeding frenzy at the hippocampal level.

When we hit our forties and are producing about half the hormones we made in our twenties, we start to feel unsure, overwhelmed, and may act more carefully or even anxiously. This is because the hippocampus is starving for some "she" and "he" attention.

A review of the literature about hormones and the hippocampus was published in an article from the Graduate School of Arts and Sciences at the University of Tokyo. The authors said that estrogen and testosterone protect brain function so completely that it is the *significant reduction of estrogen and testosterone* in middle-age that literally "initiates" dementia, Alzheimer's disease, and depression. I would add lack of sexual desire and enjoyment.

One study tracked the level of testosterone in males, the functioning of their hippocampi, and their sense of self-esteem. They found that as men age, and their testosterone levels go down, the hippocampus is less fed and less active and this correlates exactly with the degree of *less* self-esteem.

This means that a healthy hippocampus maintains healthy self esteem. Hippocampal health depends on estrogen and testosterone (and some oxytocin) signals.

You have learned that as you age, everything shrinks; your skin, the lining of your gut, and even your brain. The brain has been shown to shrink as estrogen levels lower. This is inevitable with natural aging. But if estrogen is given as replacement, this shrinkage can be *reversed*, and brain shape, function, and memory can all be improved.

Hippocampal volumes have been measured and found to be larger in postmenopausal women who are on estrogen therapy presently or in the past. The larger hippocampal volumes correlated with less anxiety, brain fog, and memory loss. And more sexual desire.

Estrogen replacement revolumizes *hippocampal shrinkage* (the true scientific term for this phenomena). The bigger and better shape of your brain, the better your entire health. This study was run by the Center for Studies on Human Stress, Douglas Hospital Research Center at McGill University.

MRIs of the brains of the women in a Norwegian study showed that those women who had taken estrogen therapy throughout menopause had a larger hippocampus. These authors also pointed out that the hippocampus is one of the structures that is *first and foremost* affected early in the progression of Alzheimer's disease. These researchers state in their article (published in January 2016 in the *Neurobiology of Aging*) that areas where hormone therapy had the greatest benefit are the same areas that are affected by Alzheimer's disease in its early stages.

Bottom line: boosting estrogen and testosterone levels increases the volume of the hippocampus and can help prevent memory loss, dementia, and depression, all while boosting the desire and pleasure of great sex. This can be done by hormone replacement, and also, in women, by the very act of enjoying sex (unprotected, in a safe relationship, so sperm and estrogens can be absorbed). It is also boosted by regular exercise, healthy diets and awakened bonking.

Studies on estrogen and the brain

If your hippocampus is not getting fed and stimulated by estrogen and testosterone, you do not feel sexy, let alone remember where your bedroom is. It's challenging to want to make love, let alone enjoy it, if you ache all over, can't think, and feel like you're 100 years old. But as Andy Dufresne said in *The Shawshank Redemption*, "Remember, Red. Hope is a good thing, maybe the best of things." Don't wait around for lack of desire, fatigue, and poor cognition to blanket your future, your dreams, and your sex life: *grasp hope*. You can and should re-volumize your hippocampus and revamp your boudoir activities.

Enter estrogen.

- In the laboratory, estrogen has been shown to *break down accumulation of beta-amyloid* and wash it out of the brain. This is the physiological *goo* that builds up in the brain and is linked with Alzheimer's disease.

- Estrogen boosts mood, increases fine motor control, and decreases pain.

- Estrogen boosts short-term memory storage and promotes a larger volume of gray matter and larger parietal and hippocampal volumes in women.

- Estrogens are *anti-inflammatory* helpers. They keep the brain free from inflammation, which is linked to headaches, brain fog, and cognitive decline. As estrogen levels go down in the blood, brain inflammatory molecules (interleukins, etc.) can rise. You want estrogens in your blood to keep a cool head.

- *Estrogen clearly protects against cognitive decline.* The Department of Neuroscience at Mount Sinai School of Medicine writes that since the 1990s, science has shown that estrogen is the main overseer of the hippocampal nerve network (structural plasticity).

- Research from the Department of Psychological Medicine, Institute of Psychiatry, King's College, London, used MRI technology and voxel-based morphometry to study the long-term effects of estrogen replacement immediately at the time of menopause. The study was run on 61 women. The findings suggest that *starting hormone replacement as close to the beginning of menopause as possible is best for slowing down gray matter deterioration.* Gray matter is where most of the nerves of the brain live and is a major component of the central nervous system.

- Research on mice certainly shows that when estrogen is given, memory is boosted. This has also been shown in humans through research at respected institutions, like McGill University Department of Psychiatry. Estrogen boosts the volume of the hippocampus. And estrogen replacement reboots the volume of the hippocampus within weeks.

- Estrogen protects nerves. It's *neurotrophic,* meaning it keeps nervous tissue healthy, especially in the brain. Thus, it protects cognition. Estrogen is so brain protective that it's been shown to protect the brain after stroke and slow down damage from the stroke in mice!

- Estrogen (and progesterone) replacement increases dendritic spine density (*dendrites* are projections from neurons that receive signals) and increases the concentration of choline acetyltransferase, which boosts production of acetylcholine, a neurotransmitter critically involved in memory. The levels of acetylcholine are markedly reduced in Alzheimer's disease as well as by regularly taking many anticholinergic medications such as antihistamines to benzos to many more. This research comes from the University of California in San Francisco where they looked at brain metabolism and volume while people took meds in real time).

- Another study from the University of California in San Francisco measured the amount of *free* form of estrogen (the form most available to the body) in 425 women and their cognitive skills. The women with higher natural forms of estrogen in their body had 70% less cognitive decline.

Smart women know this. I was part of a teaching team at a medical symposium with Dr. Pam Smith, a well-respected expert on hormones. Dr. Smith reported that estrogen is such a memory booster that she always makes sure to take her estrogen replacement on the day she lectures to keep her performance top-notch.

The fall-out from the Women's Health Initiative (WHI)

One of the most amazing studies indicating estrogen is a caretaker of brain health came out in October 2002 in one of the most respected medical journals, *Journal of the American Medical Association,* but at an unfortunate time. In July of that summer, the ill-fated Women's Health Initiative Hormone Study had just hit the headlines. At first blush, it seemed that hormone replacement (which was being tested) caused the very issues it was supposed to prevent or treat (heart disease, stroke, and cancer). This made scary headlines. Which sell.

But later re-analysis (which did not make headline news for another ten years) showed that these seemingly dire results of hormone therapy were actually due to specific issues of this singular study. The women were older. They had not been on hormones for over 10 years. They were fatter. But most importantly, the hormone therapies used were very high dosages of synthetic versions of hormones, which are the culprit for much of the damage.

Because of the scary headlines (and thus fear of litigation and disease), docs and patients, especially in the United States, stopped recommending and using hormone replacement. I wrote *Safe Hormones, Smart*

Women to let doctors and women know about this statistical fiasco and not to give up the bioidentical hormone ghost. But many missed out.

In 2014 I had the honor to interview for my blog the past president of the prestigious North American Menopause Society, a very conservative group. Dr. Steven R. Goldstein was the keynote speaker for the 62nd Annual Obstetrics and Gynecology Meeting. Dr. Goldstein has been a mover and shaker in women's health: he coined the term "peri-menopause" and invented the vaginal ultrasound evaluation standards for aging women.

Dr. Goldstein said that the *estrogen-only* "arm" (group of 8,000 women on estrogen) of the WHI, when reanalyzed, showed that estrogen replacement significantly *reduced* the risk of breast cancer. This was the opposite of what was seen in the group of ladies who were on estrogen along with *synthetic progestin*. However, breast protective action of estrogen got very little attention as it was not scary head-lines. Many younger women who could benefit from estrogen replace-ment therapy are not getting it due to continued fear and ignorance of the facts. This is so sad.

Dr. Goldstein emphasized, "There is no question that in general the harm that a lot of people associate with hormone replacement therapy is unfounded and overstated."

Timing is everything. Only a few months after that scary hormone study, a significant study came out of Utah. The Cache County Study on Memory in Aging was run by Weill Cornell Medical College and pub-lished in *Neurology* in an article that said that estrogen therapy clearly protects our brains. But it came out on the coattails of the study saying estrogen was dangerous. The "good news" link between estrogen and the brain was silenced. Up till now.

The Cache County Study followed almost 3,350 men and women who had healthy brains to start with, and over five years they tracked who developed Alzheimer's disease. Women who had been on estrogen replacement for ten years had a 50 percent reduction in developing dementia. This is very significant.

The study was continued onward for 12 more years, adding thousands of more Utahans, with various studies on dementia spinning off it. As more folks were added and tracked over time, estrogen therapy was shown to reduce dementia by at least 30% and up to 50% compared to women who had not taken it. But it had to be taken for at least ten years, and the closer the estrogen was started near the beginning of menopause, the more brain protective.

Brain health was also found to fare better if folks ate a better diet that included more fish and kept their blood pressure under control. But the best brain protection was long-term estrogen therapy (though we recommend always giving estrogen along with natural progesterone). Why would this be? As you have learned, estrogen care takes the hippocampus and brain plasticity and makes other neurotransmitters work better. And you have also learned that when women make love, sperm delivers a shot of estrogen into their blood stream via the vagina.

Testosterone and the Hippocampus

The hippocampus, in both men and women, has as many testosterone receptors as in the male prostate. This means nature wants both the male and female hippocampus to get T signals. The more testosterone there is in the bloodstream across the life of a person, the more the hippocampus is signaled and self-esteem, happiness, and memory follow.

Remember that the hippocampus has more mitochondria—energy furnaces—than any other tissue in your body. *As the hippocampus is signaled by testosterone, mitochondria are preserved.* Japanese researchers from the Takeda pharmaceutical company found that testosterone deficiency in the brain caused a significant reduction in the mitochondria, especially in the hippocampus. Most importantly, they found that these reductions in the expression of mitochondrial genes and supportive substances were reversed and recovered by testosterone replacement.

Testosterone replacement preserves and even reboots mitochondrial mass in the hippocampus!

Testosterone delivers many signals to the hippocampus, especially in the hippocampal *CA1 pyramidal neurons*, which are critical for spatial memory tasks. Testosterone replacement has been shown to keep this area of the brain younger and working better in aging mice. In other words, adding some testosterone in your hormone therapy, or made naturally by your own with regular love-making, or with exercise, or even healthy nutrient levels (such as magnesium from eating greens and taking supplements), all boost testosterone blood levels, which boost brain mitochondria numbers and function. And you maintain a sense of why you are driving down that road, or walked into a room.

This screams that how you live can affect the power of your brain. And sex is part of it, too.

Type-3 diabetes. Another aging issue of brain health is how your brain deals with sugar and insulin. Your brain (most of the time) basically eats a diet of two things: oxygen and glucose. If this fuel system goes wrong, you can't think straight. If you get insulin resistance in your brain, you get dementia. This is now referred to as type-3 diabetes of the brain.

Testosterone to the rescue! Testosterone helps promote healthy insulin signaling. This helps the brain consume its brain fuel better and boosts cognition.

Dr. R. S. Tan from the Michel E DeBakey VA Medical Center in Houston, Texas used PET scans to monitor brain function of two patients with early- and late-stage Alzheimer's disease and test the effect of testosterone replacement. The *testosterone replacement significantly improved* glucose and insulin dynamics in the brain of these patients with cognitive decline. They started to think better.

It may become malpractice to not test testosterone levels and consider T therapy in both men and women with dementia or with high risk of developing it.

This same author took 36 male patients with newly diagnosed mild-to-moderate Alzheimer's disease and gave testosterone replacement to the men with below-normal levels of testosterone. These men were then compared to the ones not given testosterone replacement. Men not on testosterone replacement had rapid deterioration of cognition. The men on the testosterone replacement had *significant improvement in cognition and spatial skills.*

Why? Testosterone protects the hippocampus and blood sugar metabolism of the brain and boosts hippocampal mitochondria!

Testosterone protects the brain by:

- Protecting the genes of the hippocampus

- Protecting genes that regulate sugar and insulin metabolism in the brain

- Keeping the brain well fed and energetic and less likely to have poorer thinking

- Remember, T is so important in the brain that there are as many receptors wanting and waiting to receive testosterone signals, in the hippocampus, in both men and women, as there are in the male prostate gland!

Hormone replacement for your brain

Hormone replacement therapy—both estrogen and testosterone in women [HRT or BHRT, bioidentical HRT] and testosterone replacement [TR] in men— reboots and rescues hippocampal function, thereby rebooting memory, confidence, and a sense of *sexiness.*

As you age, it's a smart move to get individualized testing of your hormone levels and replace hormones if necessary. Everyone is different. Some rare folks in their 80s and 90s still make enough of their own hormones to keep their sex life and brains thriving.

If you had hormonally driven cancers or are a high risk woman, you can look to testosterone and oxytocin rather than estrogen to take care of your brain. You could also get 2-methyoxyestradiol, the final metabolite of estrogen. It has no estrogenic activity at all, but is anti-inflammatory. So there are many ways to reboot hormonal brain activity even if you choose to avoid estrogen. That's why working with an in-the-know practitioner is critical for you to get the best health advice you can.

What to do?

We are living longer, but toward the end of life, more of us are living with increased disabilities. *Testing and individualized replacement of estrogen and testosterone* (and testing and balancing all our hormone family and supportive nutrients) serve to keep the brain from losing its ability to think, focus, process sugar and insulin, and for you to enjoy being inside your body and wanting to merge with another body.

Track your hormones throughout your lifetime like you do with blood sugar and cholesterol. Since our environment and food are hijacking our hormones, and doctors are seeing hormone issues in younger patients, it makes sense to get your hormones tested as early as your mid-twenties to get a baseline and then at least once a decade moving forward. This helps you and any future practitioners you work with know how to best understand your unique hormone and health picture.

If you have an underactive thyroid, you take thyroid replacement. If you have diabetes, you take insulin replacement. If you have adrenal disorders, you take physiologic dosages of cortisol. With the technologies we have today, if you are aging and slowing down, why would you not consider hormone replacement?

I want to encourage you to work with a hormone knowledgeable doc to have healthy hormonal support as you age, so your sex life and your brain won't age with you. You can slow down the Mack truck of Time. We can't completely stop aging, of course, but boy can we put on the brakes. Especially now that you have learned it is actually often more dangerous *not* to replace and balance your hormones than to age with deficient or out-of-balance hormones. And all this is backed by science.

Bonding brains

When your hormones are working right and your brain is getting its goodies, you're primed for less health woes as you age, but also for really hot sex.

Hot sex is not just about erotic fun (although that's good, too). According to the world-famous anthropologist Dr. Helen Fisher, when both of you have rewarding, mutually satisfying sex, specific areas of the brain light up that bond the two of you together. Turned-on bodies make turned-on brains. The hotter the sex, the more these brain areas are stimulated and for longer periods of time.

This "brain glue" will keep the two of you together even when the going gets tough. The more great sex you have (and the operational word here is *great* sex), especially in the honeymoon period (up to the first two years of a new relationship), and throughout life, the more your brains bond to help you stay together, come what may.

. . .

Love is not the hard part; making it stay is, and
great intimacy is a major way to accomplish that.

. . .

Love is not the hard part; making it stay is, and great intimacy is a major way to accomplish that. The better the connection, the more the bonding, the deeper and more mutual the orgasms, the easier and happier future the two of you are building.

This has been proven by brain scans of people falling in love, those living in healthy, loving relationships for years, and those in relationships that are breaking up. The relationships that work have these areas of the brain more turned on and for longer periods of time, even for years. What starts this brain glue? Intimate, deeply satisfying (awakened) hot sex for both of you.

CHAPTER 12

Give A Woman the Best
Orgasms of Her Life

*J*ohn had always thought of himself as virile and of his marriage to Jennifer as extremely successful, but over the years they found themselves making love less and less. John noticed that he just wasn't as happy about life as he had been and he had enough guts to talk to Jennifer about it. Turns out, she had been pretty sad about how their lovemaking had seemed to lose its zest, too. They were good friends, but as lovers, they were losing their bling. Without bling, some of the connection is lost in translation.

They came to me for hormone assessment, but testing showed that their hormone levels were fine. So I gently asked if they wanted to hear about awakened sex and how to do it. This means knowing where the G-spot is, and the B-spot, and healthy maneuvers meant to drive each other to great heights of pleasure. And all the while, this brings about more connection and happiness.

Boy, were they game. So I explained how to go about intimacy, based on the knowledge of how our hormones run our personalities and proclivities. I taught them exercises to get more in touch with their genitals. I explained how to touch and find each other's pleasure areas.

Within one week they came back reporting a much higher pleasure response, but no great orgasms or multiple ones. So with Jennifer's permission, I took John's hand and gave him guidance on how to stroke her, by having him do it on her arm. I showed him great ways and not so great ways. They were shocked to discover that his touch had had so little awareness, yet neither had known that or even what to call it if they had. Once his touch was changed, so was her response.

In another week they were excited to report deeper orgasms and multiple ones for both of them within the same loving-making period. They felt alive again. And connected as happy lovers. John came in with several crisp $100 dollar bills and threw down a generous tip on top of my desk. It's not often we docs get tipped!

Many of us go through life wondering what all the fuss is about sex; we don't enjoy it that much, or we meet a potential mate or even marry someone who is great on paper, but we can't connect with him or her in the boudoir. Then, sadly, this lack of mutually enjoyable intimacy erodes what could have been an amazing life together.

Great intimacy with your mate is more important than any deal in the boardroom or items checked off your to-do list. And relationships soar once you learn how to achieve *orgasmic connectivity* with each other. Just as you wouldn't be able to play golf, dance the tango, or even use Adobe Photoshop without studying and following guidelines, you also need strategies for great lovemaking and orgasms. You need to know what to do to ensure great results.

There is a lot of confusion, even in the medical literature, surrounding the female orgasm: where it is, what it is, and how to make it happen. Based on a combination of peer-reviewed science and my clinical experience of working with women and men for over forty years on everything to do with hormones, sex, and health, I will explain how to make your woman so filled with pleasure that she will want to do everything possible to make you happy in and out of the bedroom.

You will learn:

- how to give an *awakened kiss*

- how to *awaken her vagina and breasts*
- the five most sexually significant spots on the female anatomy
- foolproof protocols for multiple orgasms
- exact steps, positions, and lubricants to give your woman the most incredible orgasms of her life

The critical Mars/Venus differences

You can wish that your woman was more like you and less like a mystery. But without understanding the differences between men and women, you'll lose out on co-creating the most loyal and happy woman you could ever imagine through bringing her the most pleasure she'll ever experience. To accomplish this, you must honor the differences between testosterone and estrogen.

Women are all over the place, being emotional, verbal, and responsive to both psychological and physical cues. They are born multi-taskers. Estrogen molds women to be emotionally volatile, which keeps her unfocused on any one thing. Instead, she is attentive to a variety of cues from her surroundings.

Men are focused, solid, less verbal, and more physically oriented. They are designed to be "uni-taskers" or to see the goal and make it happen. Being so focused, men often go right to the kiss or take off the clothes and go right to the clitoris and vagina because they are testosterone-driven. They are designed to get the job done.

These actions do not work for most women.

She is *not* designed to get the job done but to be open to the *all*. Men going straight to their honey pot pushes women away emotionally and even decreases their pleasure. You need to address her "whole," not just her "hole." Attend to parts of the whole, because this is how she is wired.

She won't be able to tell you this, or even if she consciously knew any of this, most likely she would be too embarrassed to tell you to touch her all over and drive her mad by doing so.

A woman is not "given" orgasms

Initially, many women don't care as much about sex as men do. Testosterone is the more driving force of physical sex. But if a woman is awakened through a stimulating kiss, word, touch, and attitude, she will come to love and want sex as much if not more than you. I have witnessed this in my patients over and over again.

Your job is to awaken her to you and to her own body. Your behavior *encourages* orgasms to happen (along with her emotional intelligence, her ability to let go and be passionate, and her knowledge of her own body—so it's not all on you). Your behavior must be *both psychological and physical* and must address the whole of your woman, as well as the sexual points of interest.

But you cannot actually make a woman orgasm. You can perform the expert moves and conscious steps that *allow* her body to have an orgasm. Thus, a woman isn't *given* orgasms as much as placed into psychological and physical scenarios in an awakened state, which then encourages orgasms to happen.

Use it or lose it—orgasm muscle exercises

A major part of a woman's being able to have an orgasm or to heighten her orgasm is her ability to *activate the musculature of her pelvic floor* and also her belly muscles. The pubocoxcyeal muscles are found in both men and women and form a hammock-like band that stretches from the pubic bone to the tailbone, forming what is called the floor of the pelvic cavity and supporting the pelvic organs.

Just as abdominal muscles support the back, these muscles support a woman's ability to have deeper and better orgasms, so she does need to work on this till she develops an awareness of these muscles and how to flex them.

She can do this by pulling up on her muscles as if stopping a stream of urination. This recruits the muscles necessary to orgasm. If she pulls up on these muscles ten times in the morning and ten times in the evening, this gets her more in touch with her own sensations and ability to bring on an orgasm.

She can work on this on her own or with you. A man can put his finger in a woman's vagina and have her tighten her muscles around his finger in an off-and-on manner. This helps build up the capabilities of the pelvic floor muscles.

The five hot spots of the female sex anatomy

Sex is so misunderstood. We think it's either there or it isn't. Nothing can be further from the truth. How we speak, touch, and intend, our knowledge of anatomy and what is possible, and practice make it possible for us to create and maintain great sexual relations.

Here are the five hot spots on a woman's body that you need to know about for great sex:

1. The clitoris. The clitoris is the female version of the penis. It is much smaller than the penis but has almost the same number of nerve cells. However, these nerve cells are compacted into a much smaller space, so the clitoris is *astonishingly sensitive*, although its sensitivity varies from woman to woman. Some women require a light touch, almost like a breath; others need a robust touch, or they respond differently to different touches as the lovemaking continues.

Tip of the clitoral iceberg. The clitoris is more than the little rope of tissue that you feel directly with your finger. That's just the top of it. The clitoris actually has fibers that descend from that knot you feel, and these fibers wind through a hunk of tissue to land inside the anterior wall of the vagina. Where they exactly end up on the vaginal wall varies from woman to woman. These clitoral fibers in the vagina make the wall of the vagina (belly side) very sensitive and will be part of a new "pleasure button" called the "B" spot.

2. The B-spot. While you are touching the clitoris, or have your finger just inside her vagina, if you gently (operative word is *gently*) probe her lower belly above her pubic bone, you will often find another spot that, when you gently but firmly push inward and a bit downward, toward the pubic and back bones, magnifies a woman's pleasure. It is getting at clitoral fibers from outside the body and is a real turn-on.

The "B" stands both for belly and for Berkson, in that I seem to have identified this spot. I have not seen any scientific literature on it, but I have repeatedly been able to teach women and men how to find this spot and have heard that it greatly adds to sexual pleasure and diversity. When you touch the B-spot, she will suddenly have an easier time tightening all the pelvic muscles that help her focus her pleasure under your touch.

3. The A-spot. This spot is even more controversial and not as well known as the G-spot. It is located in the *anterior fornix erogenous zone* (deepest recesses of the vagina). Dr. Chua Chee Ann has said this spot boosts female lubrication and possibly female ejaculation when it is stimulated. Dr. Ann first identified this spot from his research on vaginal dryness.

4. The anus. This is an area that is also very sensitive. You can touch around it, or slightly and *very* gently into it, but it is a true sensual zone that is often ignored. You can touch it with one finger or with a two-finger hold. It is very sexy to touch this spot and another spot simultaneously. You both need to be very clean. Washing each other before sex is a great approach to foreplay. Once you touch the anus, do not touch any other areas until you clean yourself. It is critical to proceed safely.

5. The G-spot. *The G-spot is real,* and you are going to learn how to stimulate it and make your woman deliriously happy. The G-spot can orgasm separately from the clitoris. Some scientific studies say that the G-spot is made up of clitoral fibers, but a new study has identified the G-spot as a separate entity. It may be that fibers from the clitoris and the G-spot intertwine.

The G-spot controversy

In 1950 Dr. Gräfenberg described a distinct erogenous zone on the anterior wall of the vagina about one to three inches inward from the opening, which a popular book on human sexuality in 1981 dubbed the Gräfenberg or G-spot.

All the way up till May 2012, the scientific community has argued about the existence of a female G-spot. It's been hotly debated as to whether it exists or whether it's merely, as one article called it, "a gynecological UFO."

To give you an idea of the amazing controversy that unfolded, here are some typical scientific article titles that have literally filled the journals:

- "Does the G Spot Exist?" *Journal of Sexual Medicine* 2013.

- "Is the Female G-Spot Truly a Distinct Anatomic Entity?" *Journal of Sexual Medicine* 2012.

- "Review the G-Spot: A Modern Gynecologic Myth." *American Journal of Obstetrics & Gynecology* 2001.

- "Who's Afraid of the G-Spot?" *Journal of Sexual Medicine* 2010.

- "The G-Spot: Some Missing Pieces of the Puzzle." *American Journal of Obstetrics & Gynecology* 2002.

- "The G-Spot Is the Female Prostate." *American Journal of Obstetrics & Gynecology* 2002.

- "The Gräfenberg Spot (G-Spot) Does Not Exist—A Rebuttal of Dwyer PL: Skene's Gland Revisited: Function, Dysfunction and the G-Spot." *International Urogynecologica Journal* 2012.

Scouring the data, a group of researchers headed by Dr. V. Puppo published in *International Urogynecolgica* in December of 2012 and in *Clinical Anatomy* in January of 2013 that the *G-spot was bogus*. Pure Aunt Polly's snake oil.

But in May of 2012, eight to nine months *before* these negating articles came out, the G-spot was, for the *first time, absolutely verified.*

Dr. A. Ostrezenski from the Institute of Gynecology in Florida proved that the G-spot exists. His team published their findings in the *Journal of Sexual Medicine*, in an article called "G-Spot Anatomy: A New Discovery." The researchers did a distinct vaginal wall dissection on a fresh female cadaver to see if they could go in and actually identify and dissect this anatomical entity. They could. And they did.

. . .

The G-spot is an anatomical fact.

. . .

Ostreszenski's group documented that the G-spot is an anatomical fact. The G-spot turned out to be a well-delineated sac with walls that resembled fibro-connective and erectile tissues similar to what is found in the male penis. Upon cutting open this sac, small, blue, grape-like bits of the "guts" of the G-spot popped out!

A French study from 1994 called these clitoral bodies *female orgasmic nodules*. During experimental female orgasm, they were able to show characteristic nodules that appear when a woman is greatly turned on. I now think these are the grapelike parts of the belly of the G-spot.

The G-spot structure was found to have *three distinct parts*: a head, a middle belly made up of round, clustered, grape-like small bodies of tissue, and a tail. Remember, this article came out in May 2012, and since then other articles are still coming out denying that this spot exists. Science is a lot messier than most of us would like to believe.

One-finger technique for finding the G-spot

Now that the G-spot has been found, there really should be no more debate. If you want to be a great lover, you need to know how to find and stimulate it. In the beginning there may be a bit of trial-and-error, but believe me, she will be filled with awe, respect, and happiness that you believe it exists and are trying to find it to pleasure her.

Put your softened index or middle finger, well lubricated, inside her vagina. Keep your finger *soft* and *lubricated*; this is much more comfortable for her and enhances your purpose, which is her pleasure.

Gently stroke the anterior front wall (belly side) of the vagina and feel around with your finger. See if you can feel this saclike area. Some describe it as *a ridge* or *a different texture* from the other surrounding tissue or a *sensation of a spongy, slightly lumpy sack* behind that spot on the vaginal wall. Remember, you are feeling the wall of the sac that contains all three parts, and they may sit a little differently in each woman.

Once you think you have found this spot, stimulate it with your softened and lubricated finger in a curling "come to me" motion, like you are beckoning someone to come toward you.

You can stroke this area for a while and then lengthen your strokes and go all the way, slowly and gently, in and out of the vagina. Then go back to the spot. Ask your partner, "Is this spot exceptionally sexy?"

When you have found her G-spot she will gasp, "Yes!"

You can both have *fun* finding this spot. Get over embarrassment, get over the need to seem like you would know it immediately (nobody does), and encourage her to be part of your exploration and identification of this "candy button," as I like to refer to it, for educational, motivational purposes. Once she comes with you stroking her G-spot, her vagina is becoming awakened.

Strategic foreplay

For a woman, sex begins *before* entering the bedroom. Foreplay starts with how you two talk, text, and flirt throughout the day, especially in the hour or so before you start to actually make love.

Again, women are more complex, so a focused hour in the bedroom is okay once in a while, but most of the time, and especially in your first few years together, how you act toward a woman throughout the day is part of sex for her. You may be aggravated about this annoying fact about women, but there you have it. Women are all over the place, which includes the other hours of the day not spent in the bedroom, and this part counts as part of your sexiness to her.

Call her up or text her; tell her what you are intending to do to her when you make love later.

When you are together, when she's doing the laundry or at her computer, whisper in your woman's ear what you intend to do to her once you initiate sex.

Gently move her hair away from her neck, kiss her lingeringly behind her ear, and whisper what part of her turns you on and how you can't wait to touch it soon. Tell her, "I can't wait for later; it's going to be amazing."

Anticipation builds up great sexual energy in both of you. You will be surprised how much it adds to your enjoyment, too.

The more sexually charged you both are, the better the chance of having more powerful orgasms. Serve each other chocolate. Take an hour to touch each other, promising not to penetrate. Try it, and see if it's a turn-on for both of you.

Treat each other like you are candy stores, and there is so much to sample and experience. Put chocolate syrup on body parts, try ice, be creative, and come up with other ideas. Feed each other food.

An Italian study found that women eating chocolate daily had higher libidos than women who didn't eat nearly as much chocolate. The reanalysis was a bit dubious, but it can't hurt to try. Buy exotic chocolate, and try feeding each other a piece each day or for dessert after dinner.

Go to a place and pick each other up as if you were meeting for the first time. Explore and play with what might happen during the day or even the night before, to enhance what happens in the bedroom.

The operative words are *fun* and *creativity,* which boost pleasure for both of you. Yes, it's a bit of effort, but the payoff is huge!

Words and touch

Words and touch are the tools that prime the sexual pump of your lover when they are used with intention, presence, and caring. You should display confidence, authority, and patience by taking your time. That old song, women love a man with a "slow hand," says it all: take your time. Women are turned on by maleness, taking charge, and a slow firm touch filled with sensitivity and intention.

You know how women love words. Choose a few words to speak while fully focused on her. When you see how she responds, you will feel better about using words.

For example, you might say, "You taste great." Hold her wrist in your hand. Stroke her wrist slowly—*slowly*! Kiss her wrist and gaze into her eyes, whether you are at a stoplight, passing in the hallway, or on the couch. Speak slowly and seductively. "I can't wait to feel how turned on you are going to be," or, "Your scent drives me wild," or "I was remembering your great scent down there last night."

Touch connects you with her. But any touch that's not intentional, focused, and present will be annoying and distancing, not sexy. Sexy, effective touch is critical.

Awakened touch

Awakened touch is a core technique of all great lovers. It sets the scene for responsiveness and blockbuster orgasms.

Practice on yourself first. This might sound corny, but give it a try. This exercise takes five minutes and will shock you at how informative it is.

Awakened Touch Exercise

- Start with your own wrist and the inner forearm of your non-dominant hand. Put your dominant thumb (if you are right-handed, it's the thumb of your right hand) on the inside of your non-dominant wrist where a doctor would take your pulse. Gently and slowly stroke this softly as if trying to feel the tendons underneath.

- Practice touching with a sense of consciousness.

- Put your *mind's eye* under your fingers and feel what you are touching. Intentional touch is something few of us are taught or shown. I had no idea what it was until someone showed me. Now I often show my patients to help boost their intimacy.

- Now try the opposite. Touch rapidly, without intention, or in small, fast circles. Feel the difference?

I call this awakened touch because by touching with slowness, intention, and focus, you get to feel more turned on, and so does she. You are not just moving your hands aimlessly around the surface of her skin to get the job over with. Stretch outside the tendencies of your testosterone. You are exploring. You are connecting. You are having a conversation through touch, not words. I promise that the better you do this, the more pleasure for both of you.

Educate yourself about how touch can communicate *connection*, and then have fun *investigating and sharing* this with your partner. Awakened touch is very sexy for the both of you.

Awakened kiss

Only now do you really go in for the *awakened kiss*. An awakened kiss has had a buildup of your attention to the whole (arms, legs, hair, cheek); you have not just aimed at her lips straight off the bat. You have to *earn* the awakened kiss.

A woman's lips have many, many nerve endings, and playing with her lips is a huge turn-on to her. First, kiss all over the face, nose, forehead, and cheeks, and brush the lips. This creates a buildup of moving in toward her lips.

Then, finally, finally, she has felt the buildup and is moaning for you to take her lips fully. Women love a buildup. This should be obvious by now.

With full awareness, place your lips on hers and gently and slowly pry hers open. At all times, keep your tongue *soft*.

You can do any variation on a theme, but the point is to create a buildup and play with her lips—tugging, brushing, opening, sucking, and teasing.

The big turn-offs:

- Nothing turns a woman off more than a stiff, hard tongue. Yuck. Use a gentle tongue with moist, probing lips—not too wide open and not too much spit.

- A mouth that is open too wide. An open mouth is sensual and marvelous, but a mouth "too wide open," like you're trying to catch a softball, will send her fifteen feet backwards emotionally.

- Too much saliva. Yuck again. If a woman starts to feel that saliva is dripping down her lips and cheeks, this is a sexual fingernail-down-the-chalkboard kind of thing.

Gently take her lower lip in your teeth, *gently*, and tug on it.

Lip tugging, tongue against the teeth, fingers in the mouth, and touching the teeth—this is all very awakened, encouraging, and inspiring her mouth into the erogenous zone that it can be.

Make sure your breath is fresh. Halitosis is better than no breath at all, of course, but not when you want to *awaken* your partner. If she has halitosis, hand her a mint.

Everything you do to her is good for her to do right back at ya! Sex is a wonderful two-way street.

Awakened breasts

Not all women have sensitive breasts, but some have very sensitive breasts. I have discovered that some women can develop *awakened breasts*. You can stimulate her nipples (mouth, fingers, lubricate, bite not too hard but hard enough) and move from the breast to her honey spot or work both at the same time. When a woman experiences deep orgasms as her breasts are being cherished and touched, her *breasts become awakened*. When this technique is utilized over several months, a woman can actually learn to start orgasming just by having her breasts appreciated (fondled, kissed, bitten, etc.).

Exercise for *awakening breasts*

Cup her breasts with your hand with intention, gently but firmly. Tell her, "Feel your breasts enlarging with desire." Guide her awareness to her breasts and nipples coming alive, and tell her, "Feel your nipples getting hard."

Tell her to keep her awareness underneath your hand and to feel her breasts and nipples respond. This reinforces her awareness, pleasure, and knowledge of her breasts and sexual energy.

Some men are turned on by nipple stimulation, and some dislike it immensely. It's individual. But if at first it seems not a big deal, try the awakened breast technique at least over a few weeks to see if you can retrain or reframe the experience.

Varieties of Orgasms

Just as there are different types of wines and chocolate, there are *varieties of orgasms*. Neuroimaging has verified two areas of orgasm, one deeper and another more superficial, lighting up slightly different areas in the brain. But it's clear that women have various kinds of orgasms.

Studies performed with vaginal ultrasound probes while women orgasm have now proven that a woman can orgasm either from her clitoris or from her vagina. And she can orgasm more than once because she's so complex. That's the estrogen. Estrogen is complex so women are capable of more complex orgasms. You need to know where these orgasms are and how to elicit them in a grand way.

Clitoral orgasm

First off, your finger must be very lubricated, and so should her clitoris. This is true whether you are doing digital (finger) sex or oral sex. The clitoris demands *lots* of moisture, the more the better for her pleasure and a bigger orgasm (and also to achieve an orgasm faster if you only have a limited amount of time for lovemaking, like that short lunch break).

Every so often, get some moisture from her vagina (doing this is also a turn-on for her), or put your fingers in your mouth to get some of your own saliva, or in her mouth to get her saliva; just make sure to keep the clitoris moist. This makes for a very heightened experience. To not do so makes it harder for her to feel pleasure, and if it is taking a while, it might become painful for her.

You can stroke the clitoris up and down, from side to side, and in a circular motion. Different women like different touches, so tune in. If need be, *ask* about your touch so you are sure you are not doing too much or too little, but just right.

You can give her three sample strokes and ask her, "Which way do you like it best—one, two, three?" Do the same with touch. Some women like a firmer touch; some prefer softer. Ask her, "Which touch do you like best?" Then give her three choices again: soft, medium, and hard. Sometimes a woman likes a softer touch at first and then harder to finish the job. Sometimes vice versa. If a woman has been using a vibrator on herself frequently, it may take her a while to be able to come with digital (finger) stimulation.

You can take the clitoris in your mouth and gently tug and suck on it like a lollipop. This is an entirely different and pleasurable sensation for most women. Some women have such sensitive clitoral tissue that either you will have to gently introduce them to this or they won't be able to enjoy this. But in many women, this is a brand-new sensation that gives them potentially amazing pleasure. You can also alternate between varieties of clitoral stimulation methods. You can go from licking the clitoris with your tongue to sucking to touching with your fingers and back and forth.

Try two spots at once

It drives a woman mad if you have a finger on one erogenous zone and a second on another at the same time. The more spots you go after, the greater her pleasure.

- While you are stimulating her clitoris, you can use your other thumb to anchor down the top of her vaginal area in a gentle but firm downward hold toward her belly button.

- Or you can put one finger in her vagina and one on her clitoris and stimulate both areas.

- Or you can put one finger on the clitoris and another finger on her belly spot or G-spot or anus.

- Or you can keep one finger on her clitoris and the other cupping and stroking her breast.

- *Or you can use your soft and moist tongue;* oral sex on the clitoris is a huge turn-on. You can gently press her thighs against your ears and settle in. If you are uncomfortable, try a pillow under her hips to raise her genitalia to a position that is comfortable for both of you. Once you find her turn-on rhythms, you need to be consistent. Touching her anus and buttocks and thighs while you lick her is a big turn-on.

Vaginal orgasm

There was great debate over the authenticity of a vaginal orgasm compared to a clitoral one. Recent studies that placed ultrasound probes in the vaginas of orgasming women have proven that the vagina can have an orgasm that is separate from a clitoral orgasm, but is most likely from

stimulating the fibers of the clitoris that run through the anterior wall of the vagina. Still, the orgasms are coming from different places.

Not all women can do it. But once you awaken their vagina, most can experience vaginal orgasms, and they become easier and more enjoyable and leave women wanting more.

One thousand Czech women reported their vaginal orgasm consistency (from never to almost every time; only 21.9 percent never had a vaginal orgasm). This was then investigated in light of foreplay, how long the penis penetrated them, their degree of focus on vaginal sensations, what they were told in childhood and adolescence about sex, and whether they were more likely to orgasm with a longer-than-average penis.

This study found that the longer the time the penis is in the vagina and the more the woman has trained herself and feels good about focusing on this sensation (again, it's an *awareness* and *awakening* practice), the more likely she is to have a vaginal orgasm. And yes, women in this study had a better chance at a vaginal orgasm if the penis was physically longer, BUT . . .

Women do not really care about large penises! However, they do want *hard* penises because this is what turns them on and stimulates their erotic tissues.

If you guide your woman to focus on your penis inside her and what it feels like, and if her vagina is already awakened, then size and length don't matter as the G-spot has memory of orgasm, and she will have a great one.

The best position for guys who are on the smaller side is to give her a dominating experience that makes her feel like she is having sex with a man with a very large and long penis. Take the missionary position so your penis hits her clitoris. Make and keep eye contact. Make sure that your in-and-out motion is touching her clitoris and anterior wall so you are stimulating both areas of potential orgasms. This makes a woman feel as though your penis is actually several inches longer than it is. You have to make sure that, in this position, your penis is not only in her vagina but, as you stroke outward, it is also rubbing her clitoris.

Exercise: *Open Wide and Focus*

This is a powerful exercise of opening up and then focusing in, guiding your woman to be agile at both states of being. Remember, a woman is more tuned in to the whole, so this exercise strengthens her ability to focus in on a pleasure point to enable mind-boggling orgasms.

You are going to guide the woman to be in two states: *wide open* without any focus, and then turning *inward to a single point of focus*. You will guide her to be open, and then focused. This opening and focusing is a powerful tool for enhancing sexual awareness.

- While you are stimulating and stroking a woman, guide her to open up; to feel wide open; to feel open to you, to her body, to the surrounding room, and to everything. Tell her, "Feel you are wide open. Just let go and open. You have no focus. You are wide, wide open. Feel you are letting go of your body, and you are open to everything."

- Gently guide her back to one point of focus. Tell her, "Focus your mind's eye, your feelings, all on this one point." Put your finger either on her clitoris or in her vagina. Guide her. In a sexy, husky voice, ask her to move your finger to her single point of greatest pleasure. Once your finger is there, say to her, "Put all your focus under my finger. Pull all your pelvic muscles up into this one point under my finger. Focus here. If my finger is not on the most focused, pleasure-filled point, move my finger to where you feel this point is. Bring all your awareness only to this point. Together we are with you on this one incredible pleasure point."

- Stimulate this point with your finger or tongue while she focuses her attention on this point.

- Guide her to let go of this focus and to once again let go and open wide and have *no* focus. Remind her to be wide *open* once again. Open up, let go, and have no focus. In this way you go back and forth from guiding her to be *open with no focus* to then guiding her to be *focused on one point.*

- Stay on each state of being, the open-wide and the focused-in, for at least a few minutes to let her *be* with each feeling.

This exercise of *opening* and then *focusing* enhances a woman's awareness. Within several sessions, a woman becomes more awakened. Once the vagina is awakened, it becomes more and more responsive, and the woman can achieve better and more pleasurable orgasms. Soon she will have orgasms in both states as well as *between* both states, and then *continually.*

This exercise puts a woman in touch with her vagina in a way that allows her to experience more pleasure than she ever has in her life, and you will have been the man who takes her there.

This is an original technique that I developed working with thousands of women over many years. This is the first time it's been put in print. I would love to hear how this *mind-boggling, woman-opening skill* works for you and your partner.

Positions

Over the years, thousands of women have shared in the privacy of my office that they like two or three positions in a lovemaking session, but more than that makes the session feel less sexy and too physically demanding. Different positions help the man last longer and make the woman more excited and pleasured as various positions hit different pleasure spots.

Most women say that one of their favorites is the *missionary position*, in which the man lies on top of a woman. Women like this because when the man is on top, this position causes touching and stimulation of the clitoris while at the same time allowing for eye contact, which most women like. *This creates connection. Women love connection.* Remember, women are oxytocin secretors, which is the bonding hormone, so women love the connection/oxytocin sensation.

The *doggy position* is a good position for when you both are feeling somewhat naughty and in a party mood. It is a vigorous position that allows a man deeper entry, so when the man is first attempting this, he should go slowly and check with the woman to make sure she is not having pain.

Spooning is a great position as you can both touch much of each other's genitalia.

Don't stop!

Once a woman starts to breathe heavily and you feel she is on the verge of an orgasm, you need to allow her to come. You should continue the motions that you are doing consistently. If you change your position and motions too often, she will lose her focus and ability to orgasm, and it can become frustrating for both of you. You will think she takes an impossibly long time and is a pain to make love with. But if you stay steady, she'll come more quickly. Unless, of course, you want to tease her and continue sexually playing and not have her orgasm yet.

Don't ever say to a woman, "You are taking too long; you are trying too hard. God, what's your problem? Other women like it that way." These are distancing words and block her pleasure and thus your pleasure. She might be thinking, "Yikes, I am never going to open myself up and make love with him again; that comment hurt me."

When a woman is coming, you can heighten her orgasm. You can try gently tugging her hair, having another finger on another erogenous zone, dripping more saliva over her clitoris or dripping more into her vagina while orgasming. Some women like a heightened sense of domination (though make sure it is still safe), which you can achieve by holding her legs open in a controlled manner, holding her arms up over her head, or pinning her down (be careful not to make it difficult for her to breathe).

Did she come?

When a woman is truly orgasming, there will be contractions of the pelvic floor muscles that you can feel when your finger or penis is either inside her vagina or inside her anus. You will actually feel the vaginal walls contracting either around or close by your finger or penis. These contractions can't be faked.

If you are in the right place and you are not feeling at least two or more rhythmic contractions, then the woman is faking the orgasm.

In some women, there is a post-orgasm hypersensitivity of the clitoral tissues, so that now your finger causes pain rather than pleasure if it is still on the clitoris. The woman may move your hand quickly away or moan suddenly if what felt good a moment ago now feels painful. This is not set in stone for all women and can vary from woman to woman. It is another bit of data to suggest to you that a woman really had an orgasm and is not faking one.

Men can also fake orgasms.

A study in the *Journal of Sexual Research* in 2010 from the Department of Psychology and Women, Gender, and Sexual Studies at the University of Kansas investigated both men and women faking orgasms and why they did so. There were 180 male and 101 female college students; 85 percent of the men and 68 percent of the women had experienced penile-vaginal intercourse, and 25 percent of men and 50 percent of women reported pretending orgasms. Most pretended during penile penetration, but some pretended during oral sex, manual stimulation, and phone sex.

Reasons for faking orgasms were that the orgasm didn't seem to be imminent, they wanted sex to end, they wanted to avoid negative consequences, such as hurting their partner's feelings, or they wanted to obtain positive consequences, such as pleasing their partner.

Most women and men felt that women should orgasm before men and that men had the major responsibility to make women come. Once a woman has more and more orgasms and has experienced stimulation at a variety of her erogenous areas, she then can take the lead along with you. The sex dance becomes mutually rewarding.

You must learn how to play each other. It takes time to learn how to play an instrument. It will take time to learn how to play each other's bodies. This is normal. It is rarely stupendous the first time. The movies have given us this false expectation, and unfortunately in our rapid, throwaway society, often if we meet and there are no fireworks within the first few minutes, or the earth doesn't move under our feet the first time we make love, we think "Next." We miss out on a lot of possible great partners with this erroneous thinking.

Lubricants

Lubrication is a must. It's a turn on. It makes sex feel much better for her and, thus, for you. A man must always be thinking, "Is she moist enough? Time to *reslush*." You can use saliva from your mouth or her mouth, as well as the moisture from inside her vagina as lubricants.

Commercial water-based lubricants actually dry out the vagina over time. One example is KY Jelly. Polymer and oil-based lubricants will not dry out the vagina.

Some women have a condition called "dry vagina," in which she doesn't seem to get moist easily. This might make intercourse painful. It might even cause her issues outside the bedroom, such as pain and itching.

Dry vagina can occur at any age, though it is much more common during peri- and post-menopause. Estriol cream (1-3 mg) works wonders. Sometimes either testosterone or DHEA (dehydroepiandrosteone) is added. These work to make a vagina juicier within days. These are mostly scripts, but some can also be purchased over the counter.

If a woman doesn't want to use hormones or is not a candidate for them, some compounding pharmacies make creams with hyaluronic acid. Botanicals can be great healthy moisturizers, such as gingko biloba, red clover, hops, and even comfrey, which can all be put into lotions.

Creams are used nightly for two weeks; then 2-3 times a week as needed. If a woman is on hormone therapy but still suffers with a dry vagina, she can try adding PABA 100 mg twice a day (with food), which helps keep her hormone levels more "Zen" and her vagina more moist.

Awakened man

A man who has developed an awakened touch can *feel* the vagina and pelvic muscles throb and will recognize a mature, alive vagina. If he is only into his penis and not into communicating and focusing on his lover, he will not be able to feel her contractions.

The contractions and sense of an alive vagina are *subtle* but real. To the unaware finger or hand, or to people who are more into themselves than fully into each other, these may not be recognized. The man must be sensitive to feel them. The more awakened the man becomes, the more sensitive he becomes. Suddenly these contractions start to feel huge and very obvious to him. They can heighten *his* pleasure just as they are doing with her.

It's all about becoming more and more aware of ourselves, each other, and of that sizzling mutuality between partners. The operative word is *mutuality*.

Mutual oral sex is a huge turn-on for both of you.

Having your penis inside her mouth while she is in your mouth is usually extremely pleasurable for both partners. Oral sex is a wonderful way to give mutual pleasure. But some women have jaw issues, smaller mouths, or hang-ups about oral sex, so this has to be entered into gently and with respect to see how your partner feels. But with kind, adult discussion outside the bedroom, often even a shy or reluctant woman will be willing to stretch her boundaries.

Attitude

The sexiest part of your body for a woman is between your ears. If you have the right *attitude*, you will turn your woman on. A woman wants you to be manly. This makes her feel feminine. When you act manly, she feels safe, hot, and filled with pleasure. Her all-over-the-place estrogen feels like it has found a testosterone-safe haven.

Most women love to feel womanly. Nothing makes a woman feel more womanly than when you are centered in your own manliness. This means being confident, taking authority, taking the lead, but not acting scary, rude, or unsafe. If you play any fantasy scenes of dominance and power, beforehand you should have agreed on boundaries and safe words.

When you are an authoritative, take-charge, strong man (fake it till you make it if this seems foreign to you) and you treat her like a real woman, you will soon revel in the results of your actions. Your Mars will make her Venus rotate in orbit around you forever.

You can do this with the following actions:

- *Be the leader.* Don't ask for sex; make your moves to envelop and take her. It is sexy to most women to be taken in a safe way, but also in a commanding, male way.

- *Move her into positions or tell her the position you want her to move into.* Women are built to be very responsive to testosterone and testosterone-like actions, so taking charge by moving her body or telling her what you are going to do makes her feel feminine, desirable, and turned on.

- *Tell her what you are doing to her.* Telling your partner in a firm, sexy, and non-abusive manner is a big turn on.

  It is much sexier to a woman to hear you say, "I am going to touch you all over and make you very wet and then put myself way up inside you," than for you to just silently do it. Also, don't ask her ahead of time if it's okay to talk during sex. Just do it. Take charge. But you might say, "I am going to do some things during sex. If you don't like any of them, ruffle my hair and laugh."

- *To really blow a woman's mind, take charge of her orgasms.* When you say, "Don't come yet," or "I am touching you for two more minutes, and you are not allowed to come yet," or "Get ready to come soon," you show how manly you are in that you can take command of her body. This is very sexy to a woman and heightens her pleasure.

She is built at the atomic level to give. Your taking charge is allowing her to give her femaleness to you. Surrender is sexual and feminine and wired into her (but not if it's inappropriate or violent). Of course, only she can orgasm, and it's your lucky part to help her, but you can act as though you are in complete charge of even this. Life is all about ironies, and so is sex.

- *Keep teasing her.* Teasing is very sexy and pleasurable to a woman and heightens her experience of your manliness. Touch her and get her hot and bothered, but then move to another spot. Be flirtatious; be a tad outrageous. Of course, when she is close to orgasm and you both intend for her to come, that is *not* a time for teasing. That's a time to stay with the program!

- *Talk naughty.* This is a turn-on. Just do it with some taste and sophistication; don't sound like a sailor, unless you are doing a pirate sex scene and it's turning her on.

- *Let her know you are turned on by her.* The biggest turn-on is feeling that someone else is extremely turned on by us. This is huge. It's every great lover's responsibility to make the other person the object of his or her desire and attraction. So let her know how much she turns you on. Describe what you are doing as you do it. "I am holding your beautiful breasts in my hands, and I love the way your nipples feel so much that they are making me hard. I feel your nipples against my chest, and it makes me throb. I can't get enough of your scent. You turn me on more than anyone else ever has."

Of course, if you don't feel this way, that's another story, and it begs the question of why you are with her. But letting people know how much you are into them is the ultimate turn-on, and hopefully you both feel this way. That's what we want—*mutuality of attraction*. But sometimes we need to coax and bring it to the light of day if it isn't clear for you at first.

- *Stay in charge.* Sometimes women like to take charge, and this can be sexy for both of you. But most of the time, stay in charge, or if she is getting feisty, share the control panel. Manly behavior is what a woman is set up for at the atomic level. I am not referring to inappropriately aggressive behavior, which is an authentic turn off.

Back-and-forth

An article from the Centro Italiano di Sessuologia in Bologna, published in 2011 in *The European Journal of Obstetrics and Gynecologic Reproductive Biology*, discusses the female orgasm and sexual health. These experts say that if you know anatomy—where the spots are—and what you are doing, *all* physically health woman should be able to have orgasms.

Knowing how to go from one mode of pleasure to another is a turn-on for you both. Samples of some back-and-forth you might not have thought about:

- Give her oral sex, and then come up, kiss her, and put yourself in her mouth, and go back and forth that way for a while.

- Kiss her for oral sex, and then penetrate her, and then go back to oral sex; touch her clitoris or around her anus and then go back to penetration.

- Kiss and put her (very clean) toes and feet inside your mouth, penetrate her, put your toes (or fingers) in her mouth, and then go back to penetration.

- Pick two positions you and she enjoy greatly, such as missionary and spooning, and go back and forth between these two positions. Once one of you is close to orgasm in one position, go to the other and repeat.

- Get a vibrator and bring her close to orgasm, penetrate her yourself, go back to the vibrator, and then back to penetration (with penis and or finger).

- Alternate penetration by removing your penis from her vagina and moving up onto her chest, kissing her abdomen all the way up, focusing on her breasts, and bringing her close to orgasm by these maneuvers. But before she orgasms, go back down to penetration.

- Put her on her back. Put your penis gently inside her mouth, and guide her to keep her throat relaxed and open so you can go deeper than usual. Go down and penetrate her vagina, then back to her throat, and then back to her vagina.

- Move your well-lubricated finger between the G-spot and the clitoris. Stimulate one area almost to orgasm. Then go to the other and repeat. Back and forth. This will start to awaken her vagina to the possibilities and realities of multiple orgasms.

If your partner says "ouch"

If you have a partner who says that her genitals are too sensitive and any touch hurts, or if she develops infections and has tissue hypersensitivity issues, all these concerns can be dealt with by testing and addressing hormone and nutrient balance, as well as by trying a variety of the techniques discussed below. Sometimes there are underlying organic health issues that have to be addressed, such as infections that need to be treated. I have seen many women who have pain during intercourse that get healed by hormone balancing, nutrient boosting, and manual pelvic floor rehabilitation. Where there is a will, there are effective ways to enhance mutual pleasure and safety so you can both get all the health benefits and the fun.

Emotional intelligence and orgasm

Out of England comes some very fascinating sexual research from the *Journal of Sexual Medicine,* published in 2009. The article entitled "Emotional Intelligence and Its Association with Orgasmic Frequency in Women" discussed how up to 30 percent of women report having trouble orgasming. One-third of women are missing out on great sex and brain-stimulating health benefits!

The aim of their study was to investigate whether normal variations in *emotional intelligence*—the ability to identify and manage your own emotions and those of others—are associated with orgasmic frequency during intercourse and masturbation.

These researchers studied 2,035 women who completed questionnaires relating to emotional intelligence and sexual behavior. They found emotional intelligence to be positively correlated with frequency of orgasm during both intercourse and masturbation. In other words, *the more a woman feels better inside her own skin, the better she can orgasm.* The more a woman knows her own body, the better she can orgasm.

So if your woman consistently has trouble climaxing, you may want to discuss with her, outside the bedroom, how she is doing emotionally with herself.

The more a woman knows what pleases her and can then share this with her partner, the better and easier her orgasms become. Also, the more she practices having orgasms, the easier and better they are. You can try masturbating together and talking about it (or not); this can be very sexy and awakening to both of you.

C H A P T E R   1 3

Exact Steps to Make Your Man Ecstatic

*G*eorge *was a successful CPA focused on sitting in front of his computer and making money for his clients. He had no idea that sitting is the new smoking, not only bad for the heart but also for the health of his sexual organs. So George had trouble getting hard and staying hard, but he wasn't yet willing to go to a doctor or take meds or even say those words out loud.*

George started to date Donna. She was my patient and had already learned about awakened sex. She was on hormone replacement and was all ready to have a great sex life, but in waltzes George with an unwilling Willie.

Donna came back to me to talk about options since George had explained in no uncertain terms that he wasn't going to go to an expert for a problem he didn't have (all righty then)! I gave Donna exact guidelines on how to bring a man to pleasure, based on the personality, likes and dislikes of his hormones from the atoms on up. I got her to give him a nutrient formula with all the nutrients that make testosterone signaling function more optimally. I told her all the points to help George overcome his CPAed-to-death penile tissue.

Over time, with patience and exact steps, George woke up and so did their relationship. Knowledge is power.

227

Men love women who move with heightened femininity and freedom. Men love women who let them know what works and what doesn't. Men love to taste, feel, and hear your enjoyment. But at the atomic level, men are set up to *take* pleasure. In the bedroom, a woman's molecular giving is done by taking in what he is doing to you and giving him the pleasure of your pleasure. For their brain and health, frequency matters to men. Learn ways to make him want that frequency with you, and to enjoy it and long for it more and more with you, so that *you and he together* are what he equates with pleasure and love.

. . .

For their brain and health, frequency matters to men. Learn ways to make him want that frequency with you.

. . .

What you can do

Make eye contact, take his hand and put it on your body where you like to be touched.

Make the sounds of a woman who loves the way he is touching and looking at you. Don't say, "Don't do that," but make sounds and touch his penis and his buttock or wherever he likes to be touched when he does something you particularly like. He will start to sense what you like through the mutual pleasure.

The more you moan, gyrate, and radiate pleasure, the more pleasure he will get, because he knows he is giving you pleasure. Men love to give pleasure, so your main job as a great lover is to show him how much pleasure you are getting, and mean it. If you aren't getting pleasure, tell him what to do.

Don't fake it. Though there is a lot in the scientific literature about the benefits of authentic orgasms, many women fake it. But if you guide your mate, communicate with each other, and hang in there with each other, you can achieve real orgasms that give true pleasure and health benefits.

Set the scene. In the afternoon call your lover and tell him the sex day-dream you are having about him and what you want to do to him that night. At first your man may need to get used to you putting your sexual foot forward, but after a while he will find that bolder, natural, sexy behavior turns him on.

Don't think you're doing something "wrong." A great lover is *not* a master of sexual technique. It is a woman feeling sexy and natural and not worrying about technique. One of the major causes of sexual unhappiness and frustration in many women is preoccupation with sexual technique. You are not doing anything wrong; you just might be "being" wrong. You might be focused on feeling ugly and closed up, and then it isn't a matter of technique; it's your closed-up energy that won't allow the sexual energy to flow. Great sex comes easier the more natural and relaxed and mature you feel about all that is going on.

Be focused because he's focused. A man is more focused due to his testosterone template. You can touch him in a conscious, awakened manner on his face and buttocks and back, but he mostly wants genital stimulation, so appreciate that that is the way men are wired. Focus on his genitals. You can touch all over his body, but he mostly likes his genitals touched, sucked, and licked.

Ask and you shall be told. Find out what your mate likes and doesn't like. Some men like their nipples kissed and bitten; others hate it. Some men like their buttocks squeezed and slapped; others hate it. It is very sexy to a man to ask him what he likes. Say, "Do you like number one?" and gently slap his bottom. "Or number two?" and cup his balls. "Or number three?" and scratch your nails down his back. "Or all of the above?"

Shine it all back on him. The more you make him feel, hear, and experience the pleasure that you are getting and the sexiness that you are feeling, the more pleasure he will get, and he will want to make love with you and only you over and over again.

Men love oral sex

Suck on his penis and gently make circles on the head of it with your tongue while you are gently sucking up and down. Ask him about your pressure and if he would like more or less.

Try sucking his penis and licking his balls, and then change your position in a sexy manner, crawl on top of him and kiss him deeply.

Go back and forth from his mouth to his penis—up to his mouth with your whole body on his, then down to his penis, putting it in your mouth and making noises to let him know how much you are enjoying him.

The importance of body image

Focus on external appearance is our societal norm. Negative body image—the enemy of great sex—is on the rise. It's difficult to enjoy great sex when both partners don't feel the other is into them. But the more insecure you feel about YOU, the harder it is to be into the OTHER.

Joan Brumberg, author of *The Body Project*, writes that the female ideal and the pressure to achieve it have become merciless and overwhelming. Studies at Stanford University and the University of Massachusetts found that 70 percent of college women say they feel worse about their own looks after viewing images in media.

Bad body image is a widespread epidemic. In one study of college students, 74.4 percent of the *normal* weight women stated that they thought about their weight or appearance "all the time or frequently" and that they felt fat and ugly. But the women weren't alone; the study also found that 46 percent of the *normal* weight men surveyed responded the same way.

When men are *turned on*, their brain parts that relate to what they see and feel are turned on. It is not really how you look as much as how you experience yourself inside yourself that portrays yourself to him.

If you "feel" sexy and confident and relaxed, this will turn on his brain in all those areas.

You do not need to have a perfect body. But you do need to feel "perfectly comfy" inside the body you inhabit. Comfort inside yourself is contagious. Comfort inside yourself is sexy.

Self-confidence is sexier than pretty hair or a slim waistline. Looks last three minutes in the bedroom, while self-confidence lasts the whole time.

Loving your body is part of being a great lover

A positive body image means that whatever way you size your body up, it's separate from your sense of self and your confidence. Don't let worrying about your body get in the way of connecting with those with whom you are intending to share intimate time. To be a great lover, you have to get back to being a great inhabitant of your own body.

- *Stand in front of the mirror and look at the parts of yourself that you especially like.* Let that appreciation sink in. When you make love with a man, put his hands on these parts of your body.

- *Stop comparing yourself to others.* Your physiology is unique to you; get comfy with it.

- *Exercise more.* Getting physically stronger makes you inhabit your own body with more gusto, which you can share in the bedroom.

- *Spend time with others that exercise, eat well, and have good body images.* Mental wellness is contagious.

- *Practice mindfulness when it comes to negative statements about yourself.* Watch what your brain says about your body and, when you catch negative thoughts, replace them with thoughts about what you like about yourself instead.

Make sure your problem isn't physical

Elise was 40 years old and 75 pounds overweight. No doctor would take her seriously because they thought she was her own reason for being fat. She felt so badly about herself she had been isolating, crying, and had no idea how to change things around.

She became a recluse. She hid at home for several years, not leaving unless absolutely necessary. Her daughter brought her food and the world kept passing her by. Until her daughter heard me on a radio show and dragged her in.

Elise was on 14 medications. One of them, it turned out, she had started right before her rapid weight gain. It was a drug that caused rapid weight gain.

She got off that med and on hormone replacement (after being tested) and her diet got cleaned up. She lost weight. Her knees stopped hurting and she felt good enough to join a water aerobics group.

Her sex drive came back. She started flirting with the guy who mowed her lawn.. Elise's daughter and son-in-law sent me a card sharing how much they enjoyed having their mother back in their lives and at church again.

C H A P T E R   1 4

Get Out of Your Heads & Into Each Other

*T*wenty-one-year-old Sarah had just gotten married to the young man of her dreams. But she was shocked that being so in love could cause her to be such a wreck.

She had strong faith. Her church had led her to believe that sex was sinful except for having babies. Sarah was so up tight her husband couldn't enter her. Sarah and her husband knew nothing of foreplay, how to get things going, what to do for protection, and how to avoid infections. Sarah was getting recurrent bladder infections. She was having recurrent anxiety attacks. Her new husband felt like a failure. They were spiraling downward.

I had helped Sarah with a digestive issue a few years previously, so she felt safe with me. They both came in and I went over the art and science of connection. I assured them that sex, like everything else, has to be learned and practiced. I showed them the anatomy. Where the G-spot was. That we are still holy when we make love and give and receive pleasure. That being spiritual and being sexy were not opposed to each other.

They went home with hope that love was their right. And now they had the tools.

* * *

You are learning a new language, the hormone language of love.

* * *

Sex is a vocabulary. You are learning a new language, the *hormone language of love*. It may take time, but with practice, you will get it. If you ever tried to learn a new language, at first it feels awkward and difficult. But then your brain adapts and a whole new world opens up. Be ready to have your sexual/sensual connection open up, too.

It is well-established that effective sexual communication outside the bedroom is part of better pleasure and love inside the bedroom, which then helps love endure. But any communication starts with language. You have been learning how Mars is simpler and Venus is more complex and how this can be translated into sex, but even with these new tools, you still need to know how to connect. Part of the ability to sex-speak is not just in words or touch or awareness of the hard-wired biology of estrogen and testosterone, but it is also about the ability to CONNECT.

- First with "yourself" and

- Then with your "other."

Many of us misconceive that connection is *chemistry*. Immediate chemistry. We think that when we finally meet the right person, our emotional socks will roll up and down, and in mere minutes fireworks will explode. Everything will work exactly right (without much effort) because we have met exactly the right person. If you examine online dating profiles such as those found on Match.com, most people are expecting immediate chemistry.

This sets us up for failure.

Chemistry is *immediate sensation*. It is not necessarily enduring connection. It is set up on outer *wows*, like someone's looks. It can also be created by silent inner wounds. If someone else's deepest unrecognized pain from their early years of family life resonates with similar unhealed suffering in your own psyche, this meeting of "ancient wound to ancient wound" can create brain sensations of chemistry.

You can experience short-term chemistry with a person you may or may not achieve great sex with, or you may have it with people who are in no way appropriate life mates. But hot and fast chemistry is a red flag that he or she is not necessarily "the right one."

Connection, on the other hand, is building a bridge, which can be short-term with someone you don't remain with permanently, or long-term with a life partner. It may not come with bells and whistles and huge chemistry, but it is more than *just* chemistry. It starts deep and congruent and grows, if you both tend to it.

Deep connection is the basic tool for the hormone language of love. Although it takes "two to tango," it starts with YOU. The more you have connection with yourself, the more you can have it with someone else. You can then deepen it with each other. If you care about this person, this true connection can help your love endure.

On meeting someone, you may get an inner sense that this person *may* be the one. But real connection between two people comes from *learned* connection. It takes knowledge and practicing and learning about the likes and dislikes and uniqueness of this other person, and together, with mutuality, acting on this knowledge.

The more you have connected with your inner self, the easier and more meaningful and effective your connection to your other becomes.

Many of us long for connection but we have no idea how to achieve it. That is because many of us live in our heads, without deep *self-presence* and *self-awareness*.

We are disconnected from our bodies. We are disconnected from our deepest feelings. When we attempt to come together with another person, to be intimate, to maximize lasting pleasure (not just fleeting), if we are somewhat unknown and disconnected to our selves, realizing maximal mutual connection and pleasure with another person isn't easy to pull off. Take survey: http://drlindseyberkson.com/resources

Sex, great sex (and even great hugging if you want connection without intercourse) is a total experience for the mind, body, and emotions. You need to be connected on all these levels. If you are cemented inside your head, this blocks true connection.

True connection to-do's

Use the following helpful hints in your relationship with yourself as well as with your lover.

- *Admit that you might be stuck in your head.* It's okay to be nervous and uncomfortable, but the more comfortable you get, the easier it is to get out of your head.

- *Trust is a process that is not going to happen overnight.* But with practice and intention, it will happen, and the more you trust that you can get into your own body and that of your partner's, the more you will.

- *Don't wonder if you should try something; just do it, go for it, explore.* Don't worry about making mistakes. Visualize what you would love to happen, whatever that is for you: entanglement of arms, bodies moaning in pleasure. Connection of souls. See it in your head, image it in your heart, and then be open to it happening between you and your lover.

- *Say affirmations to yourself while making love and see if it helps you.* Examples, "I'm relaxed in the arms of another. I'll innately know what to do, I'm a great lover, I love sex, I'm having fun, and I'm improving brain health for both of us."

- *Sex is a self-awareness event. Focus on the parts of your body that are being touched and see how you feel.* You can practice this by touching yourself. Be creative and see what makes you feel better and have more intense pleasure. Then share your new understanding with your partner, either by words, touch, or both.

- *Sex is, of course, also a team activity.* This sounds silly to have to say, but many people make love like it is a solo activity, and the other person may as well be a living vibrator or sex toy. That is not great sex and will not light up both your brains on any MRI.

- *Less thinking and more being.* The better you connect with this other person and get out of your head, the less thinking you do. Rather, you become more "BEing-ness" than "THINKing-ness." This opens you up incredibly to more pleasure.

- *Get married to abandon,* even though you may not be married.

- *Intend to let go.* You have to get to the point where you tell your body that you trust its instincts and you are not thinking about what to do; you are feeling and doing without worrying and thinking.

- *Do. React. Let go.*

Even if this person is not the love of your life, or if it's your wife and you just had a fight earlier, or it's your honeymoon and you want to have the best sex of your life, realize that pulling off this amazing sex is all about *focusing and having an honest relationship* with that person right *here and now*.

Give him or her your undivided attention. Look in their eyes. Try to feel what they are feeling. Don't let anything else interfere, like the TV or phone or thoughts about work. Or fears about what they think about your body. Or worry about how long it will take to bring each other to orgasm. Relax into each moment of sex yoga. Be here now. Be with what you are creating with this other person.

The more attention you focus on the other person, the more you give yourself to the moment, the more comfortable you both get and the more pleasure and connection is possible.

How do you get there?

How do you become a great lover? How do you achieve great connection? Through *practice* and *patience* (and fun). It may look and feel different from your past definition of fun, but be open to the possibility that you may be about to experience a new kind of fun.

It's never too late.

Jeri and Glen, a strict Baptist couple, had been married for 43 years. They had five children, 15 grandchildren, and 10 great-grandchildren. They were pillars of the community. But between them were miles and miles of anger. They slept in separate bedrooms and fought like cats and dogs; so much so, their kids thought this was how couples related. A number of their children became adults who suffered multiple divorces.

Glen had no idea about giving a woman an orgasm. Gerry had no intention of talking about it. She felt sex was a painful terrible thing, only tolerated for baby making. She let him know she didn't like being touched, especially by him. Glen went outside the marriage for softness and sex, and when Gerry found out, her outrage got focused on his betrayal, rather than their tragedy inside the bedroom.

When I explained that sex could be enchanting and connecting, she didn't believe me. Glen had no idea he could go about things differently and achieve different, even delicious, outcomes. They came in because they both had heart disease. When I told them great sex was a great heart healer, they were so overcome, they both cried right in front of me in the office. But that got their attention.

It took a few months of individualized hormone replacement for them both, and several visits to go over anatomy, tools of awakened touch, and what connection was and how to practice it. We went over plastic models of the vagina and penis and they were amazed. Eventually, in the sunset of their lives, Gerry and Glen moved back in together, finally sharing a bedroom and a more peaceful home. The great-grandkids got entirely new messages about connection, love, and marriage.

If you are not feeling great pleasure

Go back to the steps of awakened sex: slow touch that communicates what you are tasting, smelling, and touching. Go back to the amazing human body in front of you, back to each sensation you are trying to feel. What are you feeling with your fingertips? Your lips? Your tongue? What you are seeing with your eyes?

If you still aren't *feeling*, focus on what you think the other person is feeling. Touch and try to sense what they are feeling. Taste and try to sense how they are feeling your tongue. Try to see what you perceive they are feeling. Try to enhance your own feeling by focusing on each individual aspect of your senses, or on what your mate is feeling, or on both. Take time. Tune in. Go slower. Give yourself to each small aspect of sensation and relax into it. You will be more and more awakened to pleasure and connection.

If you get scared or you don't feel anything, focus on one thing that you really like about your partner: his or her eyes, hair, lips, the smell of his or her breath, and get lost in that one focus and relax into that focus until the fear or numbness drifts away.

If none of the above works, follow the age-old advice of "Fake it till you make it." This is how we learn everything from dancing to cooking to a task at work. Smile, touch, focus, breathe (just don't fake orgasms).

Become a great actor and, before you know it, you'll start to "feel" big time. Great sex means you *feel*. You may have to practice feeling. If you don't feel yourself, focus on the other person and what they are feeling. Keep practicing. I promise it will become real for you at some point.

. . .

*You'll never want to go back to fast-food
junk sex again.*

. . .

Here is a crazy analogy for me, the veggie queen. Think of having the best burger ever. You had it at that steak house, and it was thick and juicy, made from pure steak, and it melted in your mouth. You can never go back to a cheap old burger again—or at least not with the same pleasure. *Make sex better than any burger ever.* You'll never want to go back to fast-food junk sex again.

Have fun!

Having fun is healthy, right up there with veggies and exercise. Have a clear intent to connect and for both of you to have fun. Be okay with this clear intent. Guilt is not a reality; it is a misinformed state of being you learned from others who were misinformed.

Give yourself to giggles and spontaneity. Be considerate at all times. If they don't respond, if they don't join you, if you can't get them awakened this time, don't get angry or harsh or frustrated. At this moment in time, your partner does not have enough information and experience to participate in this sexual conversation at the level you were hoping for.

Go back to patience, practice, and fun. You may need to think up some more fun ways, more awakened ways, for them to join in, but at some point, they will. When they allow what you do to light up their brains, their brains will make them open to incredible pleasure and connection, and you will have made it happen.

Intimacy Survey

After you have made love and decide that you want to continue as lovers, or deepen your relationship, you can go over this survey of intimacy together in a safe place and time. Do not take this survey in the bedroom nor immediately after lovemaking.

Rate you and your partner in the following areas:

- Communication skills
- Touch

- Kiss

- Penetration

- Dominance

- Vocal cues

- Scent

- Fun

- Creativity

Discussing these points in a non-confrontational safe place gives you data for the two Ps—*patience* and *practice*—so next time you can have an enhanced experience by learning what worked and what didn't for each of you.

If you were trying to become a great tennis player, your coach would video your playing. Later you would both go over your serve, the good and not so good ways you moved, you would focus on what worked and what didn't to improve your game. It's the same with great connecting sex, although, no, I'm not recommending you make a sex tape.

Make a pact to share this information, with love and respect. Take our survey: http://drlindseyberkson.com/resources

Self-Help Checklist For Awakened Sex

1. Physical health

The healthier you are, the easier it is to achieve great sex. Various illnesses make enjoyable sex difficult if not almost impossible, unless you take some proactive steps. Diabetes, heart disease, chronic fatigue, and adrenal dysregulation are all linked to poorer circulation and fatigue, which makes it difficult to participate in and enjoy sex.

Sex requires some cardio stamina and even muscle tone. When we don't work out and our muscles get mushy and we don't have lots of "wind," it's harder to achieve pleasure from making love. So being in shape makes for better love-making and more bennies from that love-making. But making love regularly and in an awakened manner makes for better love-making, too. It's a circle.

Any health issue can contribute to problems with ejaculation, orgasm, sexual desire, sexual performance, sexual enjoyment, and the ability and desire to "connect" intimately, sex or no sex. But remember, individual testing and rebalancing of hormones, and the nutrients and digestion they depend on, can often soften these physical woes and boost your sexual prowess even if you are ill.

2. Balanced hormone health

Balanced, healthy hormone levels are necessary for healthy sex. Both men and women need to get tested to determine if they are candidates for replacement.

If one gland or more is "ill," say your adrenal or thyroid or even if your vitamin D levels are low or abnormally functioning, then your other sex steroid hormones, such as estrogen and testosterone, may not work optimally. A knowledgeable doctor will run a thorough hormone panel in both women and men. In-depth adrenal and thyroid evaluation are a must!

Test the hormone family

- estrogens (estradiol, estrone, estriol,)

- free and total testosterone

- progesterone

- pregnenolone

- LH

- FSH (women)

- DHEA

- Cortisol (4-point 24-hour saliva test)

- fasting insulin

- vitamin D

- Thyroid panel (free T3, free T4, T3 uptake, reverse T3, TSH, TBG, as well as thyroid antibodies.)

Often a doctor will run your hormone blood levels and say you are "fine," your blood levels are within the normal range and you don't need hormone replacement. But the low normal levels may not be adequate for you to feel "great," especially sexually. You need to find a doctor that treats "you" the patient, based on your symptoms more than your laboratory levels.

You need to work with a doctor who knows your personal medical history and evaluates your hormones in light of this.

Note #1. Women have better sexual desire and enjoyment when their total testosterone is around 30 to 100 ng/dL in the blood, if not a touch higher. Some labs give reference ranges. It's important to base it on how she *feels*. Most men feel better with levels at about 700 to 800, if not closer to 1000. A woman's blood estradiol level should be 60 pg/mL if not closer to 100+ pg/mL, and her progesterone should be above 10 ng/mL. Some women feel better if their estradiol is higher, closer to 125 or 130. It is individual.

Note #2. When on hormone replacement, there is a wide set of opinions about how to "track" your hormone levels. They can be tested by blood levels, blood spot tests, saliva, and 24-urine. Different doctors use different methods. But tracking how you "feel," your set of symptoms, is the largest MUST of all. These should be monitored by a professional who specializes in hormone health and knows what they are doing.

Note #3. Men under the age of 40 should not be on testosterone replacement if they still want to have a family. Testosterone replacement can damage future fertility. Instead, replacement with HCG (human chorianic gonadrophin hormone) should be used as it does not affect fertility most of the time. Herbs, such as *Tribulus Terrestris,* can also be used. Many low T clinics do not warn men of this potential issue, or the doctors may not know about it.

3. THE TRIOLOGY—hormones, nutrients, and digestion

An effective hormone doctor understands how all *three pillars* of hormone health are essential for achieving great sex.

The sex steroid hormone pathway requires nutrients. Some patients don't need hormone replacement as much as they need nutrients. Sometimes libido, performance, and enjoyment can be "rebooted" by merely adding missing minerals and vitamins. Or clearing receptor function with receptor detoxes.

4. Healthy cholesterol levels

Cholesterol is not evil. All hormones, including sex hormones, are made from cholesterol. Statins and other cholesterol-lowering meds can lower cholesterol too much, thus lowering sex hormones. A cholesterol level of 100 to 140 will often cause a deficiency in sex hormones because there isn't a sufficient level of cholesterol for the body to manufacture hormones (such as estrogen or testosterone.) Insufficient levels of cholesterol (too low for your hormone production) can translate into less desire or ability to do the deed and poor enjoyment of sex.

5. Healthy sleep

Sleep affects all aspects of health, even hormones and sex. Insufficient sleep disrupts the family of hormones and also creates fatigue and mood issues not conducive to great intimacy. Most of us do not make much melatonin after the mid-30s or so, even if your bedroom is darkened and your computer is in the living room. This is because an aging pituitary is most likely already calcified. Melatonin replacement not only helps with sleep, it is a powerful antioxidant and caretaker of the sex steroids. I usually recommend robust dosages and types depending on the person. I also like giving it in time-release form so that it works *throughout* the night while you sleep.

6. Circulation and nitric oxide

Both men and women need great circulation to have great sex. This is why various diseases that harm circulation, like diabetes and heart disease, are frequently accompanied by sexual problems. Healthy circulation depends on the healthy release of nitric oxide. Nitric oxide is released by estrogen and testosterone. Its formation is also boosted by healthy foods (greens, arugula, beet greens, beets, nuts and seeds, and even chocolate—though "sugar-free" with stevia is better than "sugar-full." Exercise boosts circulation and so do drugs like Viagra and hormones like oxytocin, which can be helpful in both men and women.

7. Ideally, you need a mate.

You can self-satisfy, but studies show that this is not as physiologically beneficial, especially as a "brain booster," as doing it with someone you love. But if you don't have a partner, it is good to find a comfort level in satisfying yourself in the healthy spirit of "loving the one you're with."

8. Healthy sex history

Sex research has demonstrated that *healthy*, *age appropriate*, *non-addictive* self-exploration and self-masturbation in young children and teens (from five through eighteen years of age) leads to adults having more satisfying sexual interactions with other adults.

When you know how and what pleases you, you can guide your lover. Also, knowing your own body makes you more comfortable with exploring and satisfying your beloved's body.

9. Healthy lifestyle

Regular exercise, eating diverse colorful plant foods, consuming healthy non-contaminated fish meals, not smoking, and avoiding excess caffeine, alcohol, sugar, and processed foods all contribute to healthy circulation and a healthier sex life. Good fats found in seeds, nuts, avocadoes and olives boost good fat/sex functioning, too.

10. Alcohol moderation

More than two drinks in an evening tends to make someone *feel* sexier but actually makes the sexual equipment less able to *respond* and *function*. Moderate alcoholic consumption is thought to be healthy. This translates into one drink a night for a woman and two for a man. Going beyond these very moderate amounts of alcohol dims the ability to have and enjoy fabulous sex.

11. Respect each other's biology

Read the gender-bending differences between estrogen and testosterone and give each other "biological space" to be who they are wired to be. Act on these considerations *inside* the bedroom and *out*.

12. Throw guilt out the window

Learn and appreciate the benefits of sex, especially on our brains, so all guilt is gone. This opens the door to enjoying sex beyond your wildest dreams. Too many people are held back by guilt and shame. These thoughts about sex were sadly told to them when they were young, often by parents who themselves did not understand that Nature intends for us to have and benefit from amazing, enjoyable, mutual sex.

13. Develop awakened touch, kiss, and intimacy skills.

Learn exactly where, how, and why to touch each other. And honor the biological differences, translating them into winning wooing practices.

14. Seek connection.

Everyone longs to feel "chemistry" and connection is the basis for that feeling. To do anything "right," you need to practice. This is even true for connection. Practice connection and you will find chemistry.

15. Varietals of orgasms.

Discover the kinds of orgasms you both are capable of and "practice" giving them to each other.

16. Healthy *self*-relationship

A sense of self-confidence and comfort inside your body contributes to enhanced personal and mutual enjoyment. Many things contribute to feeling "comfy" inside your body suit: regular exercise, healthy diet, posture, and even hormone replacement, which can "reboot" the hippocampal volume that directly improves your sense of self.

For a woman to feel and act sexy, she needs to feel sexy and beautiful on the *inside*. A man needs to feel connected to his manliness, and this starts from the inside out for him, too.

17. Getting it right.

Sometimes you do everything right but still get the "wrong" outcomes. You may need to address specific nutrient supplementation and digestive protocols, working with a savvy nutritional expert and/or detoxification programs. (Get your copy of Self-Help Check List: http://drlindseyberkson.com/resources

Endnotes

Introduction

Psychiatr Danub. 2014 Nov;26 Suppl 1:266-8, Neurobiology of love. Cervone A.

Arch Sex Behav. 2002 Jun;31(3):289-93. Does semen have antidepressant properties?

Age Ageing. 2016 Jan 28.. Sex on the brain! Associations between sexual activity and cognitive function in older age

Nordic Psychology. 2016; V68: Factors contributing to separation/divorce in parents of small children in Sweden

Journal of Adolescent Health. 2016 Aug;59(2). Sexual function in 16 to 21 year olds in Britain

Reprod Syst Sex Disord. 2015 Dec;4(4). Clomiphene Citrate Effectively Increases Testosterone in Obese, Young, Hypogonadal Men

Chapter 1

Thanks to Ms. Angier for her kind and personal communication (Natalie Angier, *Woman: An Intimate Geography*, First Anchor Books, 2000).

Conversation shared between John and Benita Katzenellenbogen of the University of Illinois, two world experts on estrogen, and the Pulitzer Prize–winning author Natalie Angiers (*Woman: An Intimate Geography*, First Anchor Books 2000). Estrogen is up to sixty molecules referring to all the precursors, metabolites, and isomers involved in the production complexity of estrogen and the pathways through the human body.

Science. 339, 1044 (2013); Welcome to the Microgenderome.

Journal of Endocrinology. 1965 Jan:31:III–XVIL. The Early History of the Oestrogenic Hormones.

Neuroimage. 2012 Jan 16; 59(2): 1123–1131. Genetic Influences on Hippocampal Volume Differ as a Function of Testosterone Level in Middle-Aged Men.

Brain Res. 2016 Feb 15;1633:96-100. From the 90 s to now: A brief historical perspective on more than two decades of estrogen neuro-protection.

Horm Behav. 2013 Nov;64(5):755–63. Do Testosterone Declines during the Transition to Marriage and Fatherhood Relate to Men's Sexual Behavior? Evidence from the Philippines.

Horm Behav. 2002 Sep;42(2):172–81. Monthly Patterns of Testosterone and Behavior in Prospective Fathers.

Neurobiology of Aging. 2008 Jan;29(1):95–101. Hippocampal Volumes Are Larger in Postmenopausal Women Using Estrogen Therapy Compared to Past Users, Never Users and Men: A Possible Window of Opportunity Effect.

Archives of Sexual Behavior. 2011 Oct;40(5):921–6. Salivary Testosterone Levels in Men at a U.S. Sex Club.

Physiology & Behavior. 1992 Jul;52(1):195–7. Male and Female Salivary Testosterone Concentrations before and after Sexual Activity.

Chapter 2

Molecular Cellular and Endocrinology. 2004 Feb 27:215(1-2):55-62. Co-evolution of stroidogenic and steroid-inactivating enzymes and adrenal and sex steroid receptors.

General and Comparative Endocrinology. 1991 Oct;84(1):170-81. Characterization of a specific estrogen receptor in the oviduct of the little skate, Raja Erinacea.

Journal of Steroid Biochemistry. 1984 Apr:20(4B):945–53. The Early History of Estriol.

Proceeds of the National Academy of Science USA V. Feb:86:845–857; 1989/Biochemistry Identification of Androgen Receptors in Normal Osteoblast-Like Cells.

Journal of Endocrinology. 2001 Jul;170(1):27–38. Proof of the Effect of Testosterone on Skeletal Muscle.

Journal of Applied Toxicology. 1992 Feb;12(1):13–17. Hexachlorobenzene (HCB) Suppresses Circulating Progesterone Concentrations during the Luteal Phase in the Cynomolgus Monkey.

Mol Cell Endocrinol. 2012 Jul 25;358(2):208–15. doi: 10.1016/j.mce.2011.10.035. Epub 2011 Nov 9. Mechanisms of Endometrial Progesterone Resistance.

Psychoneuroendocrinology. 2014 Jan;39:194–203 Oxytocin's Impact on Social Face Processing Is Stronger in Homosexual than Heterosexual Men.

Horm Behav. 2002 Sep;42(2):172–81. Monthly Patterns of Testosterone and Behavior in Prospective Fathers.

Archives of Sexual Behavior. 2011 Oct;40(5):921–6. Epub 2010 Dec 17. Salivary Testosterone Levels in Men at a U.S. Sex Club.

Horm Behav. 1993 Dec;27(4):523-38. Roles of gonadal hormones in control of five sexually attractive odors of meadow voles (Microtus pennsylvanicus)

Chapter 3

Journal of Steroid Biochemistry. 1984 Apr:20(4B):945–53. The Early History of Estriol.

Proceeds of the National Academy of Science USA V. Feb:86:845–857; 1989/Biochemistry Identification of Androgen Receptors in Normal Osteoblast-Like Cells.

Journal of Endocrinology. 2001 Jul;170(1):27–38. Proof of the Effect of Testosterone on Skeletal Muscle.

Journal of Applied Toxicology. 1992 Feb;12(1):13–17. Hexachlorobenzene (HCB) Suppresses Circulating Progesterone Concentrations during the Luteal Phase in the Cynomolgus Monkey.

Mol Cell Endocrinol. 2012 Jul 25;358(2):208–15. Mechanisms of Endometrial Progesterone Resistance.

Horm Behav. 2013 Nov;64(5):755–63. Do Testosterone Declines during the Transition to Marriage and Fatherhood Relate to Men's Sexual Behavior? Evidence from the Philippines.

Horm Behav. 2002 Sep;42(2):172–81. Monthly Patterns of Testosterone and Behavior in Prospective Fathers.

Neurobiology of Aging. 2008 Jan;29(1):95–101. Hippocampal Volumes Are Larger in Postmenopausal Women Using Estrogen Therapy Compared to Past Users, Never Users and Men: A Possible Window of Opportunity Effect.

Archives of Sexual Behavior. 2011 Oct;40(5):921–6. Dec 17. Salivary Testosterone Levels in Men at a U.S. Sex Club.

Physiology & Behavior. 1992 Jul;52(1):195–7. Male and Female Salivary Testosterone Concentrations before and after Sexual Activity.

Psychoneuroendocrinology. 2014 Jan;39:194–203. Oxytocin's Impact on Social Face Processing Is Stronger in Homosexual than Heterosexual Men.

Arch Neurol. 1997 Feb;54(2):171-6.Language-associated cortical regions are proportionally larger in the female brain. Harasty J, Double KL, Halliday GM, Kril JJ, McRitchie DA.

Neuroimage. 2014 Oct 1;99:215-25. Sex differences in volume and structural covariance of the anterior and posterior hippocampus.

European Review of Social Psychology. 2015; 26 (1): A sociocultural framework for understanding partner preferences of women and men: Integration of concepts and evidence.

J Steroid Biochem Mol Biol. 2015 Jul;151:12-24. Origin of the response to adrenal and sex steroids: Roles of promiscuity and co-evolution of enzymes and steroid receptors.

Personal Communications with Dr. M. E. Baker M.E. Professor at Department of Medicine, 0693, University of California, San Diego, CA.

Baker M.E. Estrogen Physiology from an Evolutionary Perspective. *Reference Module in Biomedical Sciences. Elsevier.* 18-Oct-14.

Endocrinology. 2005 Jan;146(1):147-55. The androgen metabolite,

5alpha-androstane-3beta, 17beta-diol, is a potent modulator of estrogen receptor-beta1-mediated gene transcription in neuronal cells.

Endocrinology. 2013 May;154(5):1802-12. The androgen metabolite, 5 -androstane-3 ,17 -diol (3 -diol), activates the oxytocin promoter through an estrogen receptor- pathway.

Neuroethics. 2008;1:31–44. Neuroenhancement of love and marriage: the chemicals between us.

Symons D. *Darwinism and contemporary marriage.* In: Davis K, editor. Contemporary marriage. Russell Sage; New York: 1985. pp. 133–155.

Philosophy & Technology. 2012;25:561–587. Natural selection, childrearing, and the ethics of marriage (and divorce): building a case for the neuroenhancement of human relationships.

Curr Opin Psychiatry. 2013 Sep; 26(5): 474–484. Could intranasal oxytocin be used to enhance relationships? Research imperatives, clinical policy, and ethical considerations.

Psychoneuroendocrinology (2013) 38:1883. The role of oxytocin in social bonding, stress regulation and mental health: an update on the moderating effects of context and inter-individual differences.

Basic Neurochemistry: Molecular, Cellular and Medical Aspects. 6th edition. Olfaction. Stuart J Firestein, Robert F Margolskee, and Sue Kinnamon.

Br J Nutr. 2015 Jul;114(2):240-7. Dietary intakes of fats, fish and nuts and olfactory impairment in older adults.

J Neurosci. 2014 May 14;34(20):6970-84. Hyperlipidemic diet causes loss of olfactory sensory neurons, reduces olfactory discrimination, and disrupts odor-reversal learning.

Appetite. 2016 Feb 1;97:8-15. Consumption of garlic positively affects hedonic perception of axillary body odour.

J Neurochem. 2016 May 24. Estradiol-induced neurogenesis in the female accessory olfactory bulb is required for the learning of the male odor.

Physiol Behav. 2002 Mar;75(3):367-75. Pheromonal influences on sociosexual behavior in young women.

Arch Sex Behav. 1998 Feb;27(1):1-13.Pheromonal influences on socio-sexual behavior in men.

Dis Mon. 1998 Sep;44(9):421-546. Wellness in women after 40 years of age: the role of sex hormones and pheromones

Biol Reprod. 1994 Nov;51(5):920-5. Hormonal pattern of the pheromonal restoration of cyclic activity in aging irregularly cycling and persistent-estrus female rats.

J Steroid Biochem Mol Biol. 1995 Jun;53(1-6):343. Effects of steroids on the brain opioid system.

Endocrinology. 1997 Mar;138(3):863-70. Comparison of the ligand binding specificity and transcript tissue distribution of estrogen receptors alpha and beta.

J Exp Med. 1954 Sep 1;100(3):225-40. Chemical structure of steroids in relation to promotion of growth of the vagina and uterus of the hypophysectomized rat.

Endocrinology. 1979 Jun;104(6):1797-804. Evidence and characterization of the binding of two 3H-labeled androgens to the estrogen receptor.

Chapter 4

J Sex Med. 2009 Oct;6(10):2640–8. Is Sex Just Fun? How Sexual Activity Improves Health.

J Sex Med. 2009 Oct;6(10):2690–7. The Relationship between Self-Reported Sexual Satisfaction and General Well Being In Women.

J Sex Marital Ther. 2013 Oct 10. The Conditional Importance of Sex: Exploring the Association Between Sexual Well-Being and Life Satisfaction.

J Sex Res. 2013 Apr 30. "It Feels So Good It Almost Hurts": Young Adults' Experiences of Orgasm and Sexual Pleasure.

Am J Med. 2008 Apr;121(4): Initiative 295–301. Sexual Satisfaction and Cardiovascular Disease: The Women's Health Initiative.

J Sex Marital Ther. 2005 May–Jun;31(3):187–200. Are Orgasms in the Mind or the Body? Psychosocial versus Physiological Correlates of Orgasmic Pleasure and Satisfaction.

Neuroimage. 2007 Aug 15;37(2):551–60. Correlation between Insula Activation and Self-Reported Quality of Orgasm in Women.

J Sex Res. 2013 Dec 18. "Did You Come?" A Qualitative Exploration of Gender Differences in Beliefs, Experiences, and Concerns Regarding Female Orgasm Occurrence During Heterosexual Sexual Interactions.

Biol Psychol. 2006 Mar;71(3):312–5. The Post-Orgasmic Prolactin Increase Following Intercourse Is Greater Than Following Masturbation and Suggests Greater Satiety.

Arch Sex Behav. 2011 Oct;40(5):983–94. The Role of Masturbation in Healthy Sexual Development: Perceptions of Young Adults.

J Clin Epidemiol 1989;42:1227– 33. Characteristics of reproductive life and risk of breast cancer in a case-control study of young nulliparous women.

Cancer Epidemiol. 2014 Dec;38(6):700-7. Sexual partners, sexually transmitted infections, and prostate cancer risk.

Chapter 5

Arch Sex Behav. 2002 Jun;31(3):289-93. Does semen have antidepressant properties?

J Sex Med. 2010 Apr;7(4 Pt 1):1336-61. The relative health benefits of different sexual activities.

Molec Hum Reprod July 1998 Zinc, magnesium and calcium in human seminal fluid: relations to other semen parameters and fertility

Int J Androl. 1986 Dec;9(6):477-80. Zinc in human semen.

Biol Psychiatry. 2015 Oct 19. pii: S0006-3223(15)00824-0.Sex-Specific Effects of Stress on Oxytocin Neurons Correspond With Responses to Intranasal Oxytocin.

J Sex Med. 2008;5:2522–32.. Condom use for penile-vaginal intercourse is associated with immature psychological defense mechanisms.

Gerontologist 1982;22:513–8. Palmore EB. Predictors of the longevity difference: A 25-year follow-up.

BMJ. 1997 Dec 20-27;315(7123):1641-4. Sex and death: are they related? Findings from the Caerphilly Cohort Study.

J Androl. 1993:14:366-73. . Endocrinological, biophysical, and biochemical parameters of semen collected via masturbation versus sexual intercourse.

Biol Psychiatry. 2002;52:371–4. High-dose ascorbic acid increases intercourse frequency and improves mood: A randomized controlled clinical trial..

Biol Trace Elem Res. 2014 Nov;161(2):190-201. Anatomical region differences and age-related changes in copper, zinc, and manganese levels in the human brain.

Mol Neurobiol. 2016 Jan 7. Zinc Improves Cognitive and Neuronal Dysfunction During Aluminium-Induced Neurodegeneration.

J Sex Med. 2008;5:2522–32. Condom use for penile-vaginal intercourse is associated with immature psychological defense mechanisms.

Int J STD AIDS. 2008;19:590–4. Condom "turn offs" among adults: An exploratory study.

J Consult Clin Psychol 1996;64:819–28. Safer sex: Social and psychological predictors of behavioral maintenance and change among heterosexual women.

The psychobiology of human semen. In: Platek SM, Shackelford TK, eds. Female infidelity and paternal uncertainty: Evolutionary perspectives on male anti-cuckoldry tactics. New York: Cambridge University Press; 2006:141–72.

Sigma Research. Testing targets: Findings from the United Kingdom gay men's sex survey 2007. 2009. Available at: http://www.sigmaresearch.co.uk/files/report2009f.pdf (accessed November 30, 2009).

J Clin Epidemiol. 1989;42:1227– 33. Characteristics of reproductive life and risk of breast cancer in a case-control study of young nulliparous women.

Oncology. 1978;35:97–100.. Barrier contraceptive practice and male infertility as related factors to breast cancer in married women.

Folia Med. 1998;40:17–23. Breast cancer and barrier contraception: Postulated and corroborated potential for prevention.

Evolution 2001;55:994–1001. Females receive a life-span benefit from male ejaculates in a field cricket.

Annu Rev Sex Res. 2005;16:62–86.. Functional MRI of the brain during orgasm in women.

JAMA. 1953;153:1303–4. The Kinsey report. *The primitive psychology of Alfred Kinsey.* Presented as a paper at the Spring Scientific Meeting of the Maine Psychological Association, Lewiston, 1984. Available at: http://www.doctorg.com/primitive-psychology-kinsey.htm (accessed November 30, 2009).

Am J Cardiol. 2000;86:41F– 5. The mutually reinforcing triad of depressive symptoms, cardiovascular disease, and erectile dysfunction.

J Obstet Gynaecol Can. 2015 May;37(5):430-8. Association Between Use of Oral Contraceptives and Folate Status: A Systematic Review and Meta-Analysis.

Epilepsy Res. 2016 Mar;121:29-32. doi: 10.1016/j.eplepsyres.2016.01.007. Epub 2016 Jan 27. Seizure facilitating activity of the oral contraceptive ethinyl estradiol.

JAMA Intern Med. 2016 Jan 1;176(1):134-6. doi: 10.1001/jamainternmed.2015.6523. Recurrence and Mortality in Young Women With Myocardial Infarction or Ischemic Stroke: Long-term Follow-up of the Risk of Arterial Thrombosis in Relation to Oral Contraceptives (RATIO) Study.

Med Clin (Barc). 2016 Mar 4;146(5):207-11. doi: 10.1016/j.medcli.2015.10.032. Epub 2015 Dec 22. [Stroke in young adults: incidence and clinical picture in 280 patients according to their aetiological subtype].

Thromb Res. 2015 Dec;136(6):1110-5. doi: 10.1016/j.throm-res.2015.09.011. Epub 2015 Sep 16. Thromboembolism as the adverse event of combined oral contraceptives in Japan.

Cochrane Database Syst Rev. 2015 Aug 27;8:CD011054. doi: 10.1002/14651858.CD011054.pub2.

Combined oral contraceptives: the risk of myocardial infarction and ischemic stroke.

Aust N Z J Public Health. 2015 Oct;39(5):441-5. doi: 10.1111/1753-6405.12444.

Cancers in Australia in 2010 attributable to and prevented by the use of combined oral contraceptives.

Comp Biochem Physiol C Toxicol Pharmacol. 2016 Feb;180:56-64. doi: 10.1016/j.cbpc.2015.12.002. Epub 2015 Dec 10.

17 -Ethinylestradiol (EE2) treatment of wild roach (Rutilus rutilus) during early life development disrupts expression of genes directly involved in the feedback cycle of estrogen.

Comp Biochem Physiol C Toxicol Pharmacol. 2015 May;171:34-40. doi: 10.1016/j.cbpc.2015.03.004. Epub 2015 Mar 25.

17 -Ethinylestradiol can disrupt hemoglobin catabolism in amphibians.

Reprod Toxicol. 2014 Jul;46:77-84. doi: 10.1016/j.repro-tox.2014.03.001. Epub 2014 Mar 13.

Neonatal exposure to 17 -ethynyl estradiol affects ovarian gene expression and disrupts reproductive cycles in female rats.

Comp Biochem Physiol C Toxicol Pharmacol. 2016 Feb;180:56-64. doi: 10.1016/j.cbpc.2015.12.002. Epub 2015 Dec 10.

17 -Ethinylestradiol (EE2) treatment of wild roach (Rutilus rutilus) during early life development disrupts expression of genes directly involved in the feedback cycle of estrogen

Osteoporos Int. 2005 Dec;16(12):1538-44. Epub 2005 May 19. Oral contraceptive use in young women is associated with lower bone mineral density than that of controls.

Chapter 6

Dabbs, M., & Dabbs, J. M. (2000). *Heroes, Rogues, and Lovers: Testosterone and Behavior.* New York: McGraw-Hill.

PLoS One. 2013;8(1): e54120. Life History Trade-Offs and Behavioral Sensitivity to Testosterone: An Experimental Test When Female Aggression and Maternal Care Co-Occur.

Eur Heart J. 2011 Nov;32(21):2672–7. Heart Health When Life Is Satisfying: Evidence from the Whitehall II Cohort Study.

Rev Esp Cardiol. 2010;63:779–87: Vol. 63 Num.07 Differential Actions of Eplerenone and Spironolactone on the Protective Effect of Testosterone Against Cardiomyocyte Apoptosis In Vitro.

Chin Med Sci J. 2010 Mar;25(1):44–9. Sex Hormones and Androgen Receptor: Risk Factors of Coronary Heart Disease in Elderly Men.

JAMA. 2006 Mar 15;295(11):1288–99. Sex Differences of Endogenous Sex Hormones and Risk of Type 2 Diabetes: A Systematic Review and Meta-Analysis.

J Clin Endocrinol Metab. 2013 Sep 24. Beneficial and Adverse Effects of Testosterone on the Cardiovascular System in Men.

J Am Geriatr Soc. 2003 Jan;51(1):101–15; discussion 115. Testosterone Supplementation Therapy for Older Men: Potential Benefits and Risks.

Metabolism. 1996 Aug;45(8):935-9. Exercise increases serum testosterone and sex hormone-binding globulin levels in older men.

N Engl J Med. 2016 Feb 18;374(7):611-24. Effects of Testosterone Treatment in Older Men.

Int J Clin Pract. 2016 Mar;70(3):244-53. Serum testosterone, testosterone replacement therapy and all-cause mortality in men with type 2 diabetes: retrospective consideration of the impact of PDE5 inhibitors and statins.

J Steroid Biochem Mol Biol. 2003 Feb;84(2–3):159–66. The Gastrointestinal Tract as Target of Steroid Hormone Action: Quantification of Steroid Receptor mRNA Expression (AR, ERalpha, ERbeta and PR) in 10 Bovine Gastrointestinal Tract Compartments by Kinetic RT-PCR.

J Invest Surg. 2011;24(6):283–91. The Effects of Testosterone on Intestinal Ischemia/Reperfusion in Rats.

Mol Cell Endocrinol. 2008 Aug 13;290(1–2):31–43. Estrogen Synthesis in the Brain—Role in Synaptic Plasticity and Memory.

Neuroendocrinology. 2006;84(4):255–63. Local Neurosteroid Production in the Hippocampus: Influence on Synaptic Plasticity of Memory.

Neuroscience. 2006;138(3):757–64. Hippocampal Synthesis of Estrogens and Androgens Which Are Paracrine Modulators of Synaptic Plasticity: Synaptocrinology.

J Mol Neurosci. 2013 Sep 5. Brain Testosterone Deficiency Leads to Down-Regulation of Mitochondrial Gene Expression in Rat Hippocampus Accompanied by a Decline in Peroxisome Proliferator-Activated Receptor- Coactivator 1 Expression.

Essays Biochem. 2010;47:69–84. Regulation of Mitochondrial Biogenesis.

J Endocrinol Invest. 2012 Dec;35(11):947–50. Testosterone Responses to Intensive Interval versus Steady-State Endurance Exercise.

Horm Behav. 2013 Aug;64(3):477–86. Amelioratory Effects of Testosterone Treatment on Cognitive Performance Deficits Induced by Soluble A 1-42 Oligomers Injected into the Hippocampus.

Rejuvenation Res. 2013 Oct 17. Androgen Supplementation During Aging: Development of a Physiologically Appropriate Protocol.

Drugs. 2004;64(17):1861–91. Androgen Replacement Therapy: Present and Future.

Aging Male. 2004 Dec;7(4):319–24. Testosterone Therapy—What, When and to Whom?

Front Physiol. 2012 Apr 10;3:89. Testosterone and Vascular Function in Aging.

Maturitas. 2012 Feb;71(2):120–30. Depressive Disorders and the Menopause Transition.

Pharmacotherapy. 2012 Jan;32(1):38–53. Testosterone Supplementation for Hypoactive Sexual Desire Disorder in Women.

J Sex Med. 2014 Jan. Testosterone Improves Antidepressant-Emergent Loss of Libido in Women: Findings from a Randomized, Double-Blind, Placebo-Controlled Trial.

Am J Psychiatry. 2013 Dec 20. Antidepressant-Induced Liver Injury: A Review for Clinicians.

J Med Invest. 2012;59(1-2):12–27. Androgen in Postmenopausal Women.

Menopause. 2013 Sep 23. Safety of Veralipride for the Treatment of Vasomotor Symptoms of Menopause.

Maturitas. 2012 Oct;73(2):127–33. Hormonal Therapies for New Onset and Relapsed Depression during Perimenopause.

Science. 2013 Mar 1;339(6123):1084–8. Sex Differences in the Gut Microbiome Drive Hormone-Dependent Regulation of Autoimmunity.

Science. 2013 Mar 1;339(6123):1044–5. Welcome to the Microgenderome.

Mol Cell Endocrinol. 1991 Jul;78(3): C113–8. Intracrinology.

Neuroimage. 2012 Jan 16; 59(2): 1123–1131. Genetic Influences on Hippocampal Volume Differ as a Function of Testosterone Level in Middle-Aged Men

Neuroimage. 2012 Jan 16;59(2):1123-31.Genetic influences on hippocampal volume differ as a function of testosterone level in middle-aged men

Chapter 7

Neuropsychologia. 2007 Sep 20;45(12):2645–59. Toward an Understanding of the Cerebral Substrates of Woman's Orgasm.

Polski Merkuriusz Lekarski. 2012 Aug;33(194):120–3. Human Orgasm from the Physiological Perspective—Part II. [Article in Polish].

Polski Merkuriusz Lekarski. 2012 Jul;33(193):48–50. Human Orgasm from the Physiological Perspective—Part I. [Article in Polish]

Rev Med Suisse. 2006 Mar 22;2(58):784–6, 788. [The Neurophysiology of the Female Orgasm]. [Article in French].

Annu Rev Sex Res. 2004;15:173–257. Women's Orgasm.

J Sex Med. 2010 Apr;7(4 Pt 1):1336-61.The relative health benefits of different sexual activities.

Prog Urol. 2013 Jul;23(9):547–61. Anatomy and Physiology of Sexuality.

Arch Sex Behav. 2012 Oct;41(5):1145–60. A Typological Approach to Testing the Evolutionary Functions of Human Female Orgasm.

Arch Sex Behav. 2011 Oct;40(5):865–75. Are There Different Types of Female Orgasm?

Psychoneuroendocrinology. 1998 Nov;23(8):927–44. Love as Sensory Stimulation: Physiological Consequences of Its Deprivation and Expression.

BJU Int. 2013 Jul;112(2): E177-85. International Online Survey: Female Orgasm Has a Positive Impact on Women and Their Partners' Sexual Lives.

Arch Sex Behav. 2012 Oct;41(5):1145–60. A Typological Approach to Testing the Evolutionary Functions of Human Female Orgasm.

Sex Med. 2011 Dec;8(12):3500-4. New insights from one case of female ejaculation.

J Sex Med. 2014 Dec 24. Nature and Origin of "Squirting" in Female Sexuality.

Breast Cancer Res Treat. 1995 Aug;35(2):225–9. The Potential for Oxytocin (OT) to Prevent Breast Cancer: A Hypothesis

Arch Sex Behav. 1976;5:149–56.Personality correlates of male sexual arousal and behavior.

J Sex Res. 2002;39:321–5.Sexual functioning and self-reported depressive symptoms among college women.

Arch Sex Behav. 2004;33:539– 48.. Lifetime depression history and sexual function in women at midlife.

J Endocrinol. 2003. Apr;177(1):57-64. Specificity of the neuroendocrine response to orgasm during sexual arousal in men.

Neuroimage. 2013 Aug 1;76:178-82. Female orgasm but not male ejaculation activates the pituitary. A PET-neuro-imaging study.

J Sex Med. 2010 Aug;7(8):2774-81. doi: 10.1111/j.1743-6109.2009.01469.x. Epub 2009 Sep 1.Vaginal orgasm is associated with vaginal (not clitoral) sex education, focusing mental attention on vaginal sensations, intercourse duration, and a preference for a longer penis. =

J Sex Med 2008;5:2522–32. Condom use for penile-vaginal intercourse is associated with immature psychological defense mechanisms..

Chapter 8

J Clin Endocrol Metab. 1987. 64;27-31.Plasma oxytocin increases in the human sexual response.

Neuroethics. 2008;1:31–44. Neuroenhancement of love and marriage: the chemicals between us.

Behav Neurosci. 1999;113:1071–1079.The effects of oxytocin and vasopressin on partner preferences in male and female prairie voles (Microtus ochrogaster)

Nature. 2004;429:754–757. Enhanced partner preference in a promiscuous species by manipulating the expression of a single gene.

Rev Neurol. 2015 Nov 16;61(10):458-70.The social brain: neurobiological bases of clinical interest].

Brain Res. 1991;555:220–232.Localization of high-affinity binding sites for oxytocin and vasopressin in the human brain: an autoradiographic study.

Curr Opin Psychiatry. 2013 Sep; 26(5): 474–484. Could intranasal oxytocin be used to enhance relationships? Research imperatives, clinical policy, and ethical considerations.

Devi, G. (2012) *A Calm Brain: How to relax into a stress-free, high-powered life.* NY, NY, Penguin Dutton.

Physiol Behav (2003) 79:383–97. Developmental consequences of oxytocin.

J Sex Med. 2008 Apr;5(4):1022-4. Male anorgasmia treated with oxytocin.

Horm Behav. 2014 Mar;65(3):308-18.Differential effects of intranasal oxytocin on sexual experiences and partner interactions in couples.

J Physiol Sci. 2012 Nov;62(6):441-4. Oxytocin: a therapeutic target for mental disorders.

Neuroscience. 2012 Jan 3;200:13-8. Antidepressant-like effect of sildenafil through oxytocin-dependent cyclic AMP response element-binding protein phosphorylation.

J Physiol. 2007 Oct 1;584(Pt 1):137-47. Blockade of phosphodiesterase Type 5 enhances rat neurohypophysial excitability and electrically evoked oxytocin release. Estrogen *Front Endocrinol (Lausanne).* 2015 Oct 15;6:160.Oxytocin and the Estrogen Receptor in the Brain: An Overview.

J Neuroendocrinol (2004) 16:308–12.10.1111Neural pathways controlling central and peripheral oxytocin release during stress.

Arch Sex Behav. 1994 Feb;23(1):59-79. Relationships among cardiovascular, muscular, and oxytocin responses during human sexual activity.

Neuron (2012) 73:553–66.10.1016/j.neuron.2011.11.030 Evoked axonal oxytocin release in the central amygdala attenuates fear response.

Annu Rev Psychol (2014) 65:17–39.10.1146/annurev-psych-010213-115110. Oxytocin pathways and the evolution of human behavior.

Prog Neurobiol. 2009;88:127–151.Oxytocin: the great facilitator of life.

Nature Neurosci. 2004;7:1048–1054. The neurobiology of pair bonding.

Philos Trans R Soc Lond B Biol Sci. 2006;361:2173–2186. Romantic love: a mammalian brain system for mate choice.

Neuron (2012) 73:553–66.10.1016/j.neuron.2011.11.030 Evoked axonal oxytocin release in the central amygdala attenuates fear response

Metabolism (1991) 40:1226–30.10.1016/0026-0495(91)90220-Q Effect of estrogen or insulin-induced hypoglycemia on plasma oxytocin levels in bulimia and anorexia nervosa.

Proc Natl Acad Sci U S A (2001)
98:12278–82.10.1073/pnas.221451898 Increased anxiety and synaptic plasticity in estrogen receptor beta-deficient mice.

Comp Physiol. 2015 Mar 1;308(5):R360-9. Peripheral oxytocin activates vagal afferent neurons to suppress feeding in normal and leptin-resistant mice: a route for ameliorating hyperphagia and obesity.

Neurosci Lett. 1996 Apr 12;208(1):25-8.Vagus nerve mediates the increase in estrogen receptors in the hypothalamic paraventricular nucleus and nucleus of the solitary tract during fasting in ovariectomized rats.

Brain Res. 1991;555:220–232. *Neurol.* 2005;493:58–62. Romantic love: an fMRI study of a neural mechanism for mate choice.

Horm Behav. 2014 Mar;65(3):308-18. Differential effects of intranasal oxytocin on sexual experiences and partner interactions in couples.

Horm Behav. 2012;61:392–399. Modulating social behavior with oxytocin: how does it work? What does it mean?

Arch Sex Behav. 1994 Feb;23(1):59-79.Relationships among cardiovascular, muscular, and oxytocin responses during human sexual activity.

J Clin Endocrol Metab. 1987. 64;27-31. Plasma oxytocin increases in the human sexual response.

J Endocrinol. 2003. Apr;177(1):57-64.. Specificity of the neuroendocrine response to orgasm during sexual arousal in men.

Neuroimage. 2013 Aug 1;76:178-82. Female orgasm but not male ejaculation activates the pituitary. A PET-neuro-imaging study.

Biochim Biophys Acta. 2015 Oct 28. pii: S0304-4165(15)00297-4. Oxytocin opposes bacterial endotoxin - Effects on ER-stress signaling in Caco2BB gut cells.

Am J Physiol Gastrointest Liver Physiol. 2014 Oct 15;307(8):G848-62. Oxytocin regulates gastrointestinal motility, inflammation, macromolecular permeability, and mucosal maintenance in mice..

Menopause Int. 2011 Dec;17(4):120-5.Topical oxytocin reverses vaginal atrophy in postmenopausal women: a double-blind randomized pilot study.

Lab Anim (NY). 2014 Aug;43(8):260. With oxytocin, old muscles act like new.

PLoS One. 2015 Sep 24;10(9):e0137514.The Impact of Oxytocin on Food Intake and Emotion Recognition in Patients with Eating Disorders: A Double Blind Single Dose Within-Subject Cross-Over Design.

Am J Physiol Gastrointest Liver Physiol. 2014 Oct 15;307(8):G848-62. Oxytocin regulates gastrointestinal motility, inflammation, macromolecular permeability, and mucosal maintenance in mice.

Breast Cancer Res Treat. 1995 Aug;35(2):225-9. The potential for oxytocin (OT) to prevent breast cancer: a hypothesis.

Scientific Reports, 2015; 5: 16891. The structural neural substrate of subjective happiness.

Endocrinology. 1998 Dec;139(12):5015-33.

Comparative distribution of vasopressin V1b and oxytocin receptor messenger ribonucleic acids in brain

Hertoghe, T. *Passion Sex and Long Life: The Incredible Oxytocin Adventure*. Luxemburg: International Medical Books, 2010.

J Endocrinol. 2003. Apr;177(1):57-64. Specificity of the neuroendocrine response to orgasm during sexual arousal in men.

World J Urol. 2003. May;20(6):323-6.Oxytocin plasma levels in the systemic and cavernous blood of healthy males during different penile conditions.

Psychoneuroendocrinology. 2008 Jun;33(5):591-600. The acute effects of intranasal oxytocin administration on endocrine and sexual function in males.

Horm Behav. 2014 Mar;65(3):308-18. Differential effects of intranasal oxytocin on sexual experiences and partner interactions in couples.

Annales de Readaptation et de Medecine Physique, Volume 42, Number 1, January 1999 , pp. 29-32(4) Penile neuropathy. Study of 186 cases

Horm Behav. 2014 Mar;65(3):308-18. Male anorgasmia treated with oxytocin.

J Physiol. 2007 Oct 1;584(Pt 1):137-47. Oxytocin enhances brain reward system responses in men viewing the face of their female partner.

Psychoneuroendocrinology. 2014 Jan;39:74-87.Oxytocin enhances brain reward system responses in men viewing the face of their female partner.

J Sex Med. 2007 Jan;4(1):14-28. Oxytocin enhances attractiveness of unfamiliar female faces independent of the dopamine reward system.

J Neuroendocrinol. 2014 Feb;26(2):53-7.The oxytocin-bone axis.

Virchows Arch. 1994;425(5):467-72. Oxytocin inhibits proliferation of human breast cancer cell lines.

J Oncol. 2002 Aug;21(2):375-8.Oxytocin modulates estrogen receptor alpha expression and function in MCF7 human breast cancer cells.

Breast Cancer Res Treat. 1995 Aug;35(2):225-9.The potential for oxytocin (OT) to prevent breast cancer: a hypothesis. Murrell TG.

J Assist Reprod Genet. 2001 Dec; 18(12):655-9. The effect of single-dose oxytocin application on time to ejaculation and seminal parameters in men.

J Endocrinol. 2005 Sep;186(3):411–27. The endocrinology of sexual arousal.

J Endocrinol Invest. 2003 Jan;26(3 Suppl):82–6. Role of oxytocin in the ejaculatory process.

J Physiology. 2007 Oct 1;584(pt1):137-47.Blockade of phosphodiesterase type 5 enhances rat neurohypophyseal excitability and electrically evoked oxytocin release.

Nordic Psychology, Jan 12 2016 Factors contributing to separation/divorce in parents of small children in Sweden.

Medical World News from October, 1979, Dr. Jesse E. Potter

Anim Reprod Sci. 2013 Dec;143(1-4):30-7. Involvement of the orphan nuclear receptor SF-1 in the effect of PCBs, DDT and DDE on the secretion of steroid hormones and oxytocin from bovine granulosa cells.

Chapter 9

Safe Hormones, Smart Women, Berkson, DL. Awakened Medicine Press.

Postgrad Med. 2009 Jan;121(1):73-85. The bioidentical hormone debate: are bioidentical hormones (estradiol, estriol, and progesterone) safer or more efficacious than commonly used synthetic versions in hormone replacement therapy?

Menopause. 2014 Jun;21(6):612-23. Testosterone dose-response relationships in hysterectomized women with or without oophorectomy: effects on sexual function, body composition, muscle performance and physical function in a randomized trial.

Postgrad Med. 2015 Jan;127(1):1-4. Hormone abnormalities in patients with severe and chronic pain who fail standard treatments.

Pain Physician. 2012 Jul;15(3 Suppl):ES111-8. Opioid-induced hypogonadism: why and how to treat it.

Am J Med. 2013 Mar;126(3 Suppl 1):S12-8. The effect of opioid therapy on endocrine function.

Chapter 10

FASEB J. 1994 Mar 1;8(3):343–9. Modulation of Steroid Receptor-Mediated Gene Expression by Vitamin B6.

Journal of Biological Chemistry. 1992 Feb. 25; V.267(6):3819–24. Vitamin B6 Modulates Transcriptional Activation by Multiple Members of the Steroid Hormone Receptor Superfamily.

The EMBO Journal. 1988 Oct;7(10):3037–44. The N-Terminal DNA-Binding "Zinc Finger" of the Oestrogen and Glucocorticoid Receptors Determines Target Gene Specificity.

Doctor's Guide to Vitamin B6. Gaby, Alan (1984). Rodale Press, Emmaus, Pennsylvania: Rodale Press.

Reviews in Endocrine and Metabolic Disorders. 2007 Jun;8(2):161–71. Perturbed Nuclear Receptor Signaling by Environmental Obesogens as Emerging Factors in the Obesity Crisis.

British Journal of Obstetrics and Gynecology. 1998 Mar;105(3):345–51. Progesterone Resistance in Women Who Have Had Breast Cancer.

Arch Environ Health. 1991 Jul-Aug;46(4):254-5. Neurobehavioral dysfunction in firemen exposed to polychlorinated biphenyls (PCBs): possible improvement after detoxification.

Arch Environ Health. 1989 Nov-Dec;44(6):345-50. Neurobehavioral dysfunction in firemen exposed to polycholorinated biphenyls (PCBs): possible improvement after detoxification.

Cancer Prev Res (Phila). 2016 May 23. pii: canprevres.0026.2016. Effects of walnut consumption on colon carcinogenesis and microbial community structure.

Nutrition. 2015 Apr;31(4):570-7. doi: 10.1016 /j.nut.2014.06.001. Synergistic anti-tumor effects of melatonin and PUFAs from walnuts in a murine mammary adenocarcinoma model.

Nutr Neurosci. 2014 Dec 18. The effects of walnut supplementation on hippocampal NMDA receptor subunits NR2A and NR2B of rats.

Ann N Y Acad Sci. 2005 Nov;1056:430-49. Amyloid, cholinesterase, melatonin, and metals and their roles in aging and neurodegenerative diseases.

Nutrition. 2005 Sep;21(9):920-4. Melatonin in walnuts: influence on levels of melatonin and total antioxidant capacity of blood.

Toxicol In Vitro. 2014 Oct;28(7):1215-21. doi: 10.1016 /j.tiv.2014.05.015. Anti-aromatase effect of resveratrol and melatonin on hormonal positive breast cancer cells co-cultured with breast adipose fibroblasts.

Med Hypotheses. 2008 Dec;71(6):862-7. doi: 10.1016 /j.mehy.2008.07.040. Epub 2008 Sep 7. Aromatase inhibitor-induced joint pain: melatonin's role.

Breast Cancer Res Treat. 2005 Dec;94(3):249-54. Melatonin enhances the inhibitory effect of aminoglutethimide on aromatase activity in MCF-7 human breast cancer cells.

Int J Cancer. 2006 Jan 15;118(2):274-8. Melatonin inhibits the growth of DMBA-induced mammary tumors by decreasing the local biosynthesis of estrogens through the modulation of aromatase activity.

Br J Cancer. 2007 Sep 17;97(6):755-60. Inhibitory effects of pharmacological doses of melatonin on aromatase activity and expression in rat glioma cells.

Chapter 11

Age Ageing. 2016 Mar;45(2):313-7. Sex on the brain! Associations between sexual activity and cognitive function in older age.

Int J Geriatr Psychiatry. 2014 May;29(5):441-6. Cognitive functioning and its influence on sexual behavior in normal aging and dementia.

Am J Alzheimers Dis Other Demen. 2013 Dec;28(8):759-62..The impact of mild cognitive impairment on sexual activity.

Neuroimage. 2012 Jan 16;59(2):1123-31. Genetic influences on hippocampal volume differ as a function of testosterone level in middle-aged men.

JAMA. 2002 Nov 6;288(17):2123-9. Cache County Memory Study Investigators.

Annals of the New York Academy of Sciences. 2010 Aug;1204:104–12. Estrogen and the Aging Brain: An Elixir for the Weary Cortical Network.

Int Rev Psychiatry. 2013 Dec;25(6):673-85.The Cache County Study on Memory in Aging: factors affecting risk of Alzheimer's disease and its progression after onset.

Neurology. 2012 Oct 30;79(18):1846-52. Hormone therapy and Alzheimer disease dementia: new findings from the Cache County Study..

Science Daily, 29 August 2000. University Of California, San Francisco. "Women's Natural Estrogen Levels Help Protect Against Cognitive Decline, UCSF/VA Study Says."

Neurobiol Aging. 2015 Sep;36(9):2555-62. Perimenopausal hormone therapy is associated with regional sparing of the CA1 subfield: a HUNT MRI study.

Front Neuroendocrinol. 2016 Jan 12. pii: S0091-3022(16)30002-4. Estrogens, inflammation and cognition.

Proceedings of the National Academy of Sciences, 2015; 201522150. Rapid increases in immature synapses parallel estrogen-induced hippocampal learning enhancements.

Annals of the New York Academy of Sciences. 2010 Aug;1204:104–12. Estrogen and the Aging Brain: An Elixir for the Weary Cortical Network.

Clinical Calcium. 2013 Aug;23(8):1141–50. Role of Androgen in the Elderly. Modulation of Synaptic Plasticity by Brain-Synthesized Androgens. [Article in Japanese]

Maturitas. 2012 Nov;73(3):186–90. Estrogens, Hormone Therapy, and Hippocampal Volume in Postmenopausal Women.

Journal of the American Medical Association. 2002 Nov 6;288(17):2123–9. Hormone Replacement Therapy and Incidence of Alzheimer Disease in Older Women: The Cache County Study.

Neurology. 2001 Dec 26;57(12):2210–6. Hormone Replacement Therapy and Reduced Cognitive Decline in Older Women: The Cache County Study. Cache County Study Group.

Frontiers in Neuroendocrinology. 2008 Jan;29(1):88–113. Brain Aging Modulates the Neuroprotective Effects of Estrogen on Selective Aspects of Cognition in Women: A Critical Review.

Journal of Molecular Neuroscience. 2014 Apr;52(4):531–7. Brain Testosterone Deficiency Leads to Down-Regulation of Mitochondrial Gene Expression in Rat Hippocampus Accompanied by a Decline in Peroxisome Proliferator-Activated Receptor-Coactivator 1 Expression.

Neurobiol Aging. 2008 Jan;29(1):95–101. Hippocampal Volumes Are Larger in Postmenopausal Women Using Estrogen Therapy Compared to Past Users, Never Users and Men: A Possible Window of Opportunity Effect.

J Cereb Blood Flow Metab. 2011 Feb;31(2):413–25. Estrogen Enhances Neurogenesis and Behavioral Recovery after Stroke.

J Urol. 2000 Apr;163(4):1333–8. Altered Synaptic Transmission in the Hippocampus of the Castrated Male Mouse Is Reversed by Testosterone Replacement.

Aging Clinical and Experimental Research. 2013 Jun;25(3):343–7.

Testosterone Effect on Brain Metabolism in Elderly Patients with Alzheimer's Disease: Comparing Two Cases at Different Disease Stages.

Climacteric. 2009 Aug;12(4):301–9. Effects of Estrogen Therapy on Age-Related Differences in Gray Matter Concentration.

Chapter 12

This chapter includes portions I coauthored for a book on erectile dysfunction (*Reviving Mr. Happy: prepublication*).

Int Urogynecol J. 2012 Dec;23(12):1665–9. Does the G-Spot Exist? A Review of the Current Literature.

Clin Anat. 2013 Jan;26(1):134–52. Anatomy and Physiology of the Clitoris, Vestibular Bulbs, and Labia Minora with a Review of the Female Orgasm and the Prevention of Female Sexual Dysfunction.

ISRN Obstet Gynecol. 2011;2011:261464. Anatomy of the Clitoris: Revision and Clarifications about the Anatomical Terms for the Clitoris Proposed (without Scientific Bases).

Int Urogynecol J. 2012 Dec;23(12):1665–9. Does the G-Spot Exist? A Review of the Current Literature.

J Sex Med. 2012 May;9(5):1355–9. G-Spot Anatomy: A New Discovery.

J Sex Med. 2010 Aug;7(8):2774–81. Vaginal Orgasm Is Associated with Vaginal (Not Clitoral) Sex Education, Focusing Mental Attention on Vaginal Sensations, Intercourse Duration, and a Preference for a Longer Penis.

J Sex Med. 2012 Dec;9(12):3079–88 Women Who Prefer Longer Penises Are More Likely to Have Vaginal Orgasms (but Not Clitoral Orgasms): Implications for an Evolutionary Theory of Vaginal Orgasm.

Eur J Obstet Gynecol Reprod Biol. 2011 Jan;154(1):3–8. Embryology and Anatomy of the Vulva: The Female Orgasm and Women's Sexual Health.

J Sex Med. 2009 Jul;6(7):1930–7. Emotional Intelligence and Its Association with Orgasmic Frequency in Women.

Gynecol Obstet Fertil. 2007 Jan;35(1):3–5. Clitoris and G Spot: An Intimate Affair.

Gynecol Obstet Fertil 2007;35:3–5. Clitoris and G spot: a fatal connection.

Contracept Fertil Sex. 1994 Nov;22(11):727–30. Female Orgasmic Nodules.

J Sex Med. 2006 May;3(3):476–82. Chocolate and Women's Sexual Health: An Intriguing Correlation.

Chapter 13

Brumberg, J. J. (1997). The Body Project: An Intimate History of American Girls. New York: Random House.

Cash, T. (1997). The Body Image Workbook: An 8-Step Program for Learning to Like Your Looks. Oakland: New Harbinger Publications.

Hutchinson, M. G. (1985). Transforming Body Image. Freedom: Crossing Press.

Kilbourne, J. (1999). Can't Buy My Love: How Advertising Changes the Way We Think and Feel. New York: Touchstone Books.

Pope, H. G., Phillips, K. A., & Olivardia, R. (2002). The Adonis Complex: The Secret Crisis of Male Body Image. New York: Touchstone Books.

The Journal of Sex Research, 2016; 1 DOI: 10.1080/00224499.2015.1137854

Chapter 14

The Journal of Sex Research, 2016; 1 DOI: 10.1080/00224499.2015.1137854. What Keeps Passion Alive? Sexual Satisfaction Is Associated With Sexual Communication, Mood Setting, Sexual Variety, Oral Sex, Orgasm, and Sex Frequency in a National U.S. Study.

Resources

Work with me!

I can work with you as a solo consultant or along with my medical team, or have me work along with your own doctors. I specialize in *reversing the irreversible*, and the strategic, safe uses of hormone, nutritional and gut boosting protocols.

Contact:

Berkson Health

Email: info@drlindseyberkson.com

Websites:

DrLindseyBerkson.com
BodyMindHormones.com
HormoneDisruption.com
SexyBrainSystem.com

Click here for FREE Food-gasm recipe booklet from Dr. Berkson's kitchen. http://drlindseyberkson.com/sexybrain/

Go to SexyBrainSystem.com for more information.

To order **OxySpray** (Over-The-Counter Oxytocin Nasal Spray)

CareFirstPharmacy.com

Phone: (918) 994-1400

(presently not shipped to all states)

Index

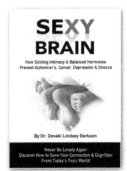

Made in the USA
Middletown, DE
07 May 2023

30175417R00176